A Guide to the Identification of Prey Remains in Otter Spraint

by JWH Conroy, J Watt , JB Webb & A Jones

Contents

A guide to the identification of prey remains in otter spraint 3rd edition
By J.W.H. Conroy, J. Watt, J. Webb and A. Jones

Published by The Mammal Society

The Mammal Society
Registered Charity No. 278918
Registered Office:
The Mammal Society
2B Inworth Street
London SW11 3EP

ISBN 0 906282 551

This booklet replaces earlier versions by JWH Conroy, J Watt, JB Webb and A Jones *A Guide to the Identification of Prey Remains in Otter Spraint* (1993, Occasional Publication No. 16) and by JB Webb *Otter Spraint Analysis* (1980, Occasional Publication No. 13)

Front cover illustration by Ruth Pollitt
Drawings on page 4 by Guy Troughton, from *How to Find and Identify Mammals* 2nd edition by Sargent, G and Morris, P 1999 The Mammal Society
All other drawings by Anna Jones

Typesetting and printing by SP Press, Units 1 & 2, Mendip Vale Trading Estate, Cheddar Business Park, Cheddar, Somerset BS27 3EL

Introduction

One of the most important aspects of animal ecology is knowing what individuals eat. This is particularly true for otters, *Lutra lutra*, where recent research has shown a strong relationship between the availability of food, and the distribution and survival of the species (Kruuk 1995; Kruuk *et al.* 1987, 1991, 1993). Knowledge of otter diet is clearly important for otter conservation.

An examination of the otter's diet shows that it can be very varied and contains a vast number of species, including fish, mammals and birds (See Herfst 1984; Chanin 1985; Mason & Macdonald 1986 for details). This key, however, is restricted primarily to identifying fish species eaten from bones or bone remains recovered from spraints (faeces), and covers only the more important species taken by otters in British rivers and seas.

Since The Mammal Society's publication of *Otter Spraint Analysis* (Webb 1980), our understanding of otter ecology has increased dramatically, particularly in coastal areas, such as Shetland (see Kruuk *et al.* 1991 and Kruuk 1995 for detailed references). The original volume was restricted to primarily freshwater prey. Later Watson (1978, 1986) produced keys which contained descriptions of many marine species.

Because of the importance of amphibians, particularly frogs, in the diet at certain times of the year (Weber 1989), their bones are shown in Appendix 1.

Detailed descriptions of mammal and bird remains can be found in more specialised keys, including Day 1966; Brunner & Coman 1974; Debrot *et al.* 1982; Watt *et al.* 1992.

Methods of determining diet

There are three methods of determining what otters eat.

1. **Direct observations of individuals feeding.** By far the best method, because it allows us to see exactly what otters are eating - the prey species and its size. It can also give an indication of individual feeding preferences. The principal drawback to this method is that, in most areas, otters are solitary, nocturnal, secretive and rare animals, making such observations difficult. Where it has been possible, e.g. diurnal otters in Shetland, the results of such studies have been very rewarding (Kruuk & Moorhouse 1990).

However, in most instances it is necessary to use indirect methods such as:

2. **Analysis of stomach contents.** The remains in the stomachs and intestines of dead otters are examined. Otters are protected in Britain and throughout much of Europe, so that it may be difficult to obtain large enough samples from animals found dead in one area to make a meaningful study.

3 **Analysis of spraints (faeces).** Like most carnivores, otters have a fairly rapid digestion and their spraints contain the remains of undigested parts of their prey, such as bones, scales, feathers and hair; these can be used to identify what has been eaten.

Spraint analysis is the most common method of assessing diet, but its use has several problems. These have been described by Putman (1984) and are not discussed in detail here other than to say that the faeces contain only the undigested remains. Soft-bodied or very large animals, where only the flesh is eaten, leave little or no undigested remains. Consequently these animals will be under-represented in any sample. At best spraint analysis gives an index of diet and cannot usually give information on the actual numbers of prey eaten, except rarely, e.g. single-element bones such as the atlas vertebra. (Details of how to calculate diet composition are given in Appendix 2).

Suitability of otter spraints in diet analysis

Spraints are ideal for studying diet because they are:

1 readily identified in the field by their characteristic appearance and smell. They vary in colour from grey to brown or black, are generally cylindrical in shape and up to 5 cm long. Large spraints often break into two or three parts. Initially they are wet and slimy but dry out when exposed to air. The smell is variously described as fishy, musty, or fungus-like and is readily recognised. The only other faeces that might be mistaken for otter's are those of American mink (*Mustela vison*). However, mink faeces tend to be smaller and thinner than otter spraints, and they are often more twisted, pointed at the ends and their smell is also more offensive (Fig. 1).

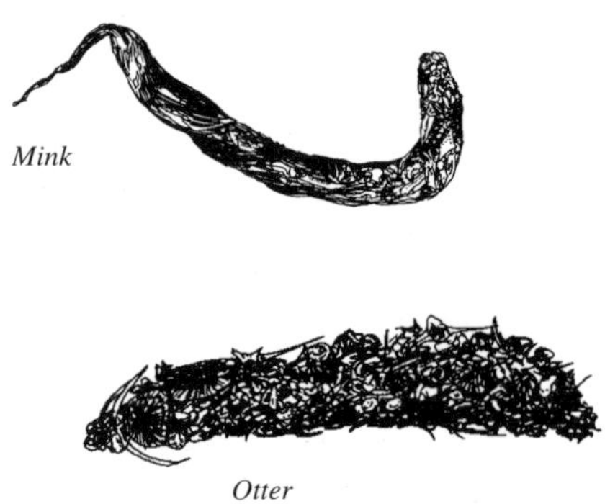

Figure 1: *A comparison of the scats of otters and American mink.*

2 usually easy to find, being regularly deposited out of, but usually near, water throughout the otter's range. Sprainting places which have been used over long periods of time, are easily recognised in the field. The faeces add nitrogen to the immediate surroundings, making the sites very conspicuous. For example, rocks have green tops, while grassy areas such as knolls tend to be bright green with more luscious vegetation than the surrounding area. Some areas, particularly on the coasts, which have been heavily used over a number of years, may be bare of any cover; the continual addition of nitrogen eventually kills all plant growth and exposes the soil, which is often covered with small bones.

Otters tend to choose prominent objects as spraint sites. In freshwater habitats these might include large boulders in midstream, protruding tree roots, ledges or banks under bridges, stream junctions and places where otters regularly leave or enter the water. In marine habitats spraints are found most frequently on rocky coasts (Conroy & French 1985, 1987), at the mouths of streams, on otter runs and, at certain times of the year, at the entrances to holts. Freshwater pools and lochans near the coast are often favoured as sprainting places.

In many parts of their range, however, sprainting on land may be seasonal (Conroy & French 1991), making it more difficult to find spraints at times when their numbers are low. Spraint sites also tend to be much larger in the marine environment, with several being found within a small area, each often containing many spraints. For example, in the space of 12 months on a small rocky ledge at the base of a cliff in Shetland, the number of sites varied from a low of zero in summer to 15 in winter and the number of spraints ranged from zero to over 250.

Collection and storage of spraints

If spraints are being regularly collected over a long period of time, it is best to identify the key sprainting sites in an area and use them as the collection points rather than check random stretches of river or coast. This approach makes much better use of the time spent in the field collecting spraints, which even on rivers with healthy otter populations can mean hours of walking and searching. The minimum number of spraints which needs to be collected will depend on the variety of species eaten by the otters and the degree of accuracy required by the researcher. For most freshwater systems within the UK ten to 15 spraints will probably give a very good indication of the main prey, while in the marine habitat around 25 spraints are needed (Mason & Macdonald 1980; pers. obs.).

Throughout the whole process of collecting, preparing and subsequently identifying the prey in the spraints, care should be taken to ensure only minimum damage to the bones. These may be very brittle and easily broken, often resulting in the loss of important diagnostic characteristics such as spines.

Most spraints are relatively easy to collect and can be picked up by hand (it is recommended that rubber gloves be worn to do this). However, very old and dehydrated spraints are likely to crumble when picked up by hand and are of limited use. In such cases a small spoon should be used for collection. Small fresh spraints should be collected in the same way. Whenever possible, old spraints should not be used in any detailed study of diet because it is usually not possible to tell how long ago they were deposited. Where spraints are stuck to rocks or roots they can often be removed with the help of a small penknife.

Once collected, each spraint should be placed in a separate marked container; for this small polythene bags are best, labelled with details of the date and where found. If analysis is not to begin immediately, the spraints should be frozen. They can be kept for long periods of time in this condition.

Preparation of spraints for analysis

Details of how to prepare spraints for subsequent analysis are well documented elsewhere (see Jenkins *et al.* 1979). Here we summarise the procedure.

1. Before the contents of any spraint can be examined, they have to be freed from the dark slimy mucilaginous materia, which hold them together. This is achieved by soaking individual spraints in a saturated solution of a biological washing agent. The solution with the spraint is shaken and left over night.

2. Once the bones have been freed, the solution is then emptied onto a sieve of 0.5mm mesh and gently washed to remove any remaining mucus and soil particles. The undigested remains can then be removed from the sieve and placed on filter paper.

3. There are now two courses of action. The bones can either be identified immediately, or else they can be air dried and then identified. In some instances the bones have been oven dried, but we would urge against this because such drying can result in shrinkages of as much as 10% of the bones' size (pers. obs.).

Identification

The bones and other remains are usually only a few millimetres long, so identification is best achieved by using a binocular microscope (x10 magnification). Often, however, large bones can be easily identified by the naked eye or with a lens. This is often useful in the field. If a spraint with only a few large bones is found, collection may not then be necessary.

In addition to having good keys, identification is greatly enhanced by using as a reference a collection from known fish species. The value of such a collection is that bones from spraints can be compared directly with bones that have come from a previously identified species.

The choice of bones to be used in the key

The bones in otter spraints are usually intact, making the choice for prey identification wide. We have, however, concentrated on only two elements – vertebrae and, in some instances, the premaxillae.

Not surprisingly, the most commonly occurring identifiable bones in spraints are vertebrae, owing to the large number present in a single fish. They are the principal bones described here and have a number of advantages over other bones:

- they can be used to estimate prey size (Casteel 1976; Wise 1980);
- even when damaged they are often easily recognisable;
- as there are many vertebrae in an individual fish, the likelihood of recovering a well-preserved specimen is good.

Other recognisable elements of fish appearing in spraints include prevomers, jaw, pharyngeal and opercular bones, hyomandibulars, post-temporals and palatines. With the exception of the first named, these are all paired bones and can be used to estimate a minimum number of fish in the spraint. Although many of these bones can be identified to the species, jawbones were considered to have a number of advantages over the others for inclusion in this key.

Being directly involved in feeding, jaws have undergone much modification and adaptation, providing the variety of form required for easy specific identification and so they may be readily distinguished from other elements found in spraints. Of the four jawbones - premaxillae, maxillae, dentaries and articulars - most premaxillae offer the advantage of robustness and ease of description and have been included here for a number of species.

A key to dentaries and articulars from a wide variety of fish is found in Izquierdo (1988). The vertebrae and premaxillae of those fish which form an important part of otter diet are described. For further guidance on the identification of premaxillae and vertebrae of a much larger number of marine species, see Watt *et al.* (1992).

Vertebrae

The vertebral column of fish

The vertebral column of fish (Fig. 2) is made up of numerous segmentally arranged vertebrae, extending from the base of the skull to the tail. The precise form of each varies, depending upon its position along the column. No two adjacent bones are identical. They can be divided into three groups - anterior abdominal, thoracic and caudal vertebrae (Fig. 3).

Anterior abdominal vertebrae

These are characterised by centra bearing a fused neural spine with no laterally projecting processes. The first vertebra attaches to the basioccipital at the base of the skull and is called the atlas. This bone and the axis (the one immediately posterior to the atlas) are often strongly compressed. The length of successive bones increases slightly along the column.

Thoracic vertebrae

These bear transverse processes (the parapophyses) on their centra, to which the ribs are attached. In the first few, they arise high up the centrum, but on successive ones their bases are situated lower down and the processes themselves are inclined more steeply downwards. There is little variation in the lengths of individual thoracic vertebrae from a single fish.

Caudal vertebrae

The transition from thoracic to caudal vertebrae is marked by the fusion of the two transverse processes to form the haemal spine. In some species, e.g. salmon, this fusion is via a connecting strut of bone between the processes, while in many others, including the gadids and flatfishes, the processes themselves come together forming an arch.

Choice of vertebrae for identification

Since vertebrae vary to such an extent within an individual fish, we have focussed principally on the caudal vertebrae and specifically on the more anterior ones.

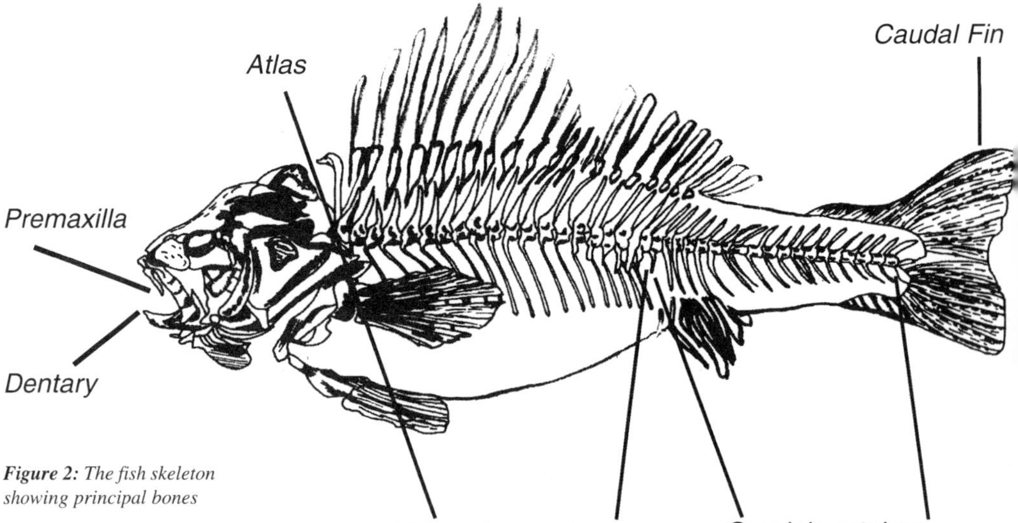

Figure 2: *The fish skeleton showing principal bones*

Figure 3: The main bones of the fish vertebral column

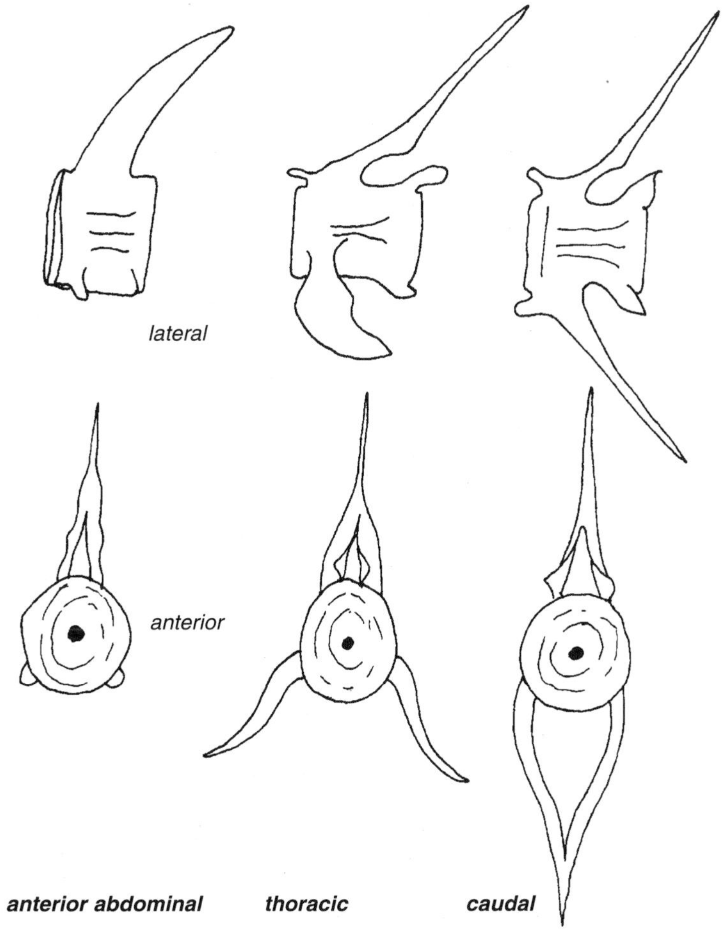

The criteria used in this choice are twofold. Firstly, at least until very close to the tail fin, caudal vertebrae show a more limited range of variation than the anterior abdominal and thoracic bones. Secondly, the fused processes of caudal vertebrae are less prone to breakage than the unfused processes of thoracic vertebrate, resulting in a greater likelihood of finding well-preserved specimens.

Once practised at recognising caudal vertebrae, it is usually quite straightforward to identify thoracic vertebrae from the same species - caudal and thoracic vertebrae from the same species exhibit many similar features.

For some prey, including the more important freshwater prey, salmonids and eels, the thoracic vertebrae are also described.

Variations within caudal vertebrae

While caudal vertebrae exhibit fewer variations than thoracics, they are far from identical within an individual, varying in two principal ways along the length of a fish:

- moving posteriorly along the column, the haemal and neural spines become more strongly inclined;
- the centra change in size and shape. In most species, the more posterior centra are relatively narrow compared to those situated anteriorly.

Structure of caudal vertebrae and nomenclature

Fig. 4 shows a generalised caudal vertebra. The spool-like **centrum** is concave at both ends. Running longitudinally through its centre is the **spinal foramen**, which is all that remains of where the notochord was found. Its size relative to the diameter of the centrum can be important, often providing clues for the identification of isolated centra. In lower forms of fish, such as salmonids and clupeids, it is large and conspicuous, while in higher forms it is reduced.

Dorsally the **neural spine** provides attachment for swimming muscles and, in many species, support for the fin pterygiophores. The **neural arch** provides protection for the spinal cord. Nerves exit the arch either via foramina if the base of the neural spine is broad, or through open grooves if it is not. The presence or absence of **neural foramina** is useful diagnostically. Ventrally the **haemal spine** is formed from the fusion of the parapophyses. It too provides muscle attachment and fin support, while the **haemal arch** gives protection to the large blood vessels running along the underside of the centra and, in some species, the swim bladder.

Arising both anteriorly and posteriorly are a number of further projections, the **zygapophyses**, those anterior are termed **prezygapophyses** (the anterior zygapophyses of Watson (1978)), those posterior are the **postzygapophyses**. Both the pre- and postzygapophyses of adjacent vertebrae overlap to provide strength and rigidity to the vertebral column. Their presence, size and shape vary between groups and species and they are, therefore, valuable diagnostically. They are most conspicuously developed in strongly swimming species such as scads, mackerels and tunnies.

The vertebrae of some species, including many flatfish and conger eels, bear lateral projections or **apophyses** on either side in the midline of the centrum. In the flatfishes these are normally more strongly developed on the upper (eyed) side than on the lower (blind) side. The function of the apophyses is as skeletal support for the muscle (Ford 1937).

Figure 4: *Caudal vertebra showing principal features described in the text*

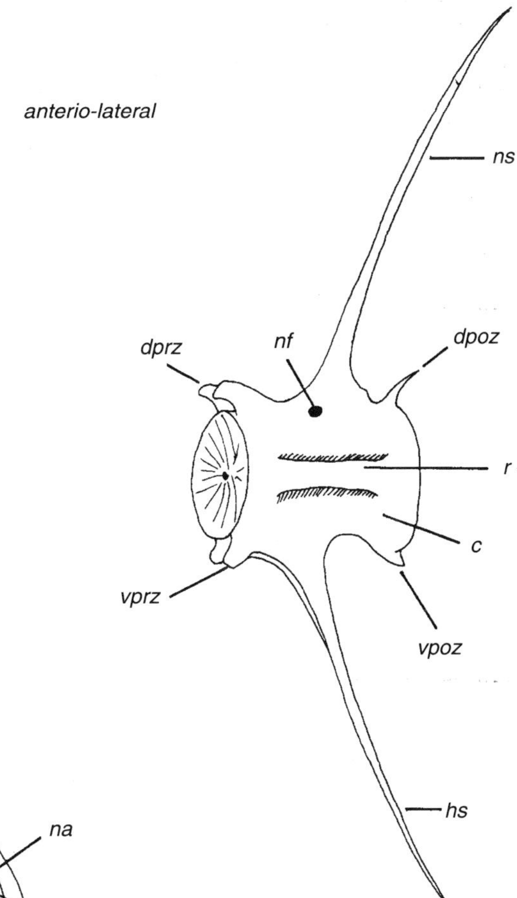

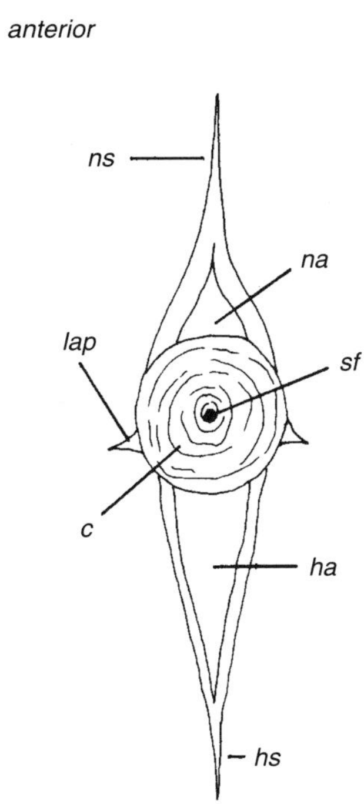

c - centrum
r - rib
dprz - dorsal prezygaphophyses
dpoz - dorsal postzygapophyses
vprz - ventral prezygapophyses
vpoz - ventral postzygapophyses
ns - neural spine
hs - haemal spine
na - neural arch
ha - haemal arch
nf - neural foramen
sf - spinal foramen
lap - lateral apophyses

Premaxillae

The premaxillae are a pair of bones that form the anterior margin of the upper jaw (Fig. 5). They consist of a curved part, the **ramus**, which constitutes the edge of the upper jaw and is generally blunt near its anterior, where it curves medially towards its opposite number. The anterior surface may be grooved or notched for the insertion of fibrous tissues or cartilage between the opposing premaxillae. When present this groove is the **anterior premaxillary cleft**. The ventral or ventro-medial surface of the ramus is usually toothed (Fig. 5c).

Three processes arise from the dorsal surface of the ramus, the most anterior being the **ascending process**. In fish with protrusible jaws, such as the Cottidae, these can be very long, allowing the premaxilla to slide forwards and outwards as the jaws are extended. Immediately behind is the **articular process**, the medial surface of which articulates with the anterior end of the maxillary. These are the **anterior processes** and are usually divided by the **interprocess notch**. The third process arising from the ramus, **the post maxillary process**, projects upwards and in most species lies against the medial surface of the maxilla. It is usually a thin sheet of bone, which is frequently damaged or absent in premaxillae found in spraints or stomachs.

In most species, excluding flatfish, the right and left premaxillae are mirror images.

Notes about the key

Many of the principal species that appear in the diet of otters in the UK are listed in the key. There are fish species not detailed here which are important to otters in some parts of the country; these can be either added to the key, or recognised from bones in a reference collection. The taxonomy follows Miller and Loates (1997) and each fish species is categorised as being freshwater (F), marine (M) or both (FM) to aid identification.

Unless otherwise stated the vertebrae described are always caudal.

In some cases, the bones of a family of fishes are similarly shaped, e.g. the Cyprinidae. In this instance only one species is described in detail, the other species are then listed at the end of the section. Where two species of fish from different families are similarly shaped, details of the differences between them are described.

Where data are available on the relationship between vertebra size and fish length, the relevant equations are given and their sources are listed. Where more than one calculation is available, these are listed. The equations described in the text to calculate fish length from their vertebrae differ depending upon who made the calculation; only in some instances are sample sizes and correlations are listed.

The size of the vertebrae vary from species to species so the size of the bones in the sketches should NOT be used as a comparison between species.

Note: In the text

FL	=	Fish length:
VW	=	Vertebra width:
VL	=	Vertebra length:
r	=	correlation coefficient
n	=	number of fish in the sample
cf.	=	compare with

__Figure 5:__ Premaxilla, showing principal features described in the text

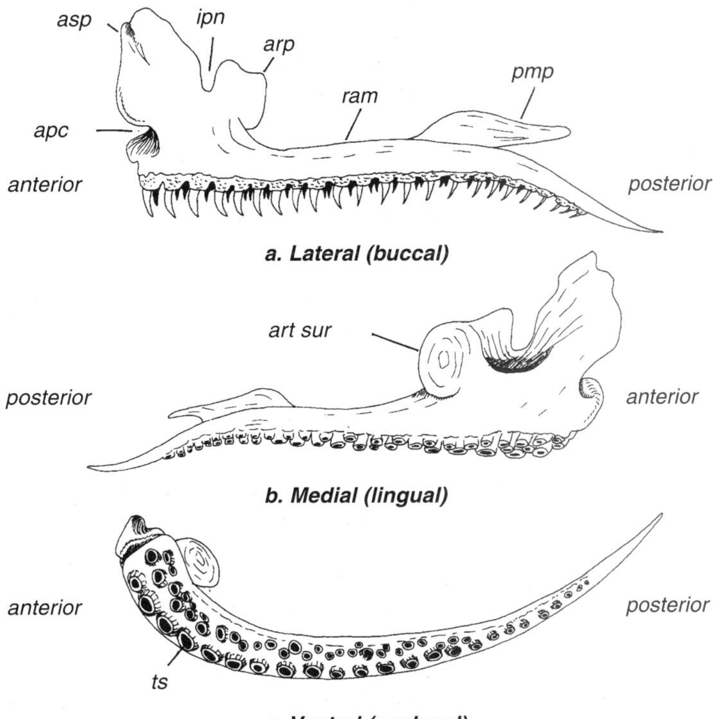

apc - anterior premaxillary cleft
asp - ascending process
arp - articular process
art sur - articular surface
pmp - postmaxillary process
ram - ramus
ipn - interprocess notch
ts - tooth socket

Key to Fish Vertebrae

To assist with identification, species that are found only in freshwater systems are marked (F); those that occur in both marine and freshwater habitats are marked (FM).

	Bone characteristics	Species	Go to
1	Vertebra has no spines		2
	Vertebra has spines		3
2	Centrum honeycombed - with ribs	**Salmonid (thoracic; FM)**	
	Centrum honeycombed - no ribs	**Pike (F)**	
3	Vertebra triangular when viewed end-on	**Stickleback (FM)**	
	Vertebra not triangular		4
4	Neural spine - (roughly) central		5
	Neural spine not central		23
5	Neural & haemal spines are short, near vertical and flattened laterally	**Pipefish**	
	Not like this		6
6	Dorsal prezygapophyses present		7
	Dorsal prezygapophyses absent		33
7	Dorsal prezygapophyses - small or may be absent		8
	Dorsal prezygapophyses - prominent		12
8	Lateral apophyses - prominent	**Flatfish**	
	Lateral apophyses - none		9
9	Vertebra translucent, papery and usually large	**Lumpsucker**	
	Vertebra not translucent		10
10	Haemal spine – broad-based (much longer than neural spine)	**Sea snail**	
	Haemal spine - thin		11
11	Haemal & neural spines thin & curved centrum honeycombed	**Salmonid (FM)**	

12	Dorsal prezygapophyses inclined:		
	horizontally		13
	vertically		16
13	Vertebra chunky		14
	Vertebra not chunky		15
14	Neural spine curves vertically		
	Dorsal prezygapophyses		
	extend beyond centrum	**Bullrout/Sea scorpion**	
	Single thick lamellar keel		
	Spines short and swept back	**Bullhead**	
15	Single prominent keel	**Butterfish**	
16	Centrum narrow-waisted		17
	Centrum not narrow-waisted		18
17	Narrow-waisted centrum		
	- shiny appearance		
	- broad base to spines		
	- hole in base of haemal spine	**Stickleback (FM)**	
18	No lamellar ribs present	**Stone loach (F)**	
	Lamellar ribs present		19
19	Single rib		
	- bone usually pale green	**Eelpout**	
	More than one rib		20
20	Ribs thin		21
	Ribs thick		22
21	Two/three thin ribs	**Yarrell's blenny**	
22	Two thick ribs (occasionally one)		
	long ventral prezygapophyses		
	long thin spines with bases of		
	unequal size	**Perch (F)**	
23	Neural spine - anterior		24
	Neural spine - posterior		29

24	Dorsal prezygapophysis - very small or absent		
	Vertebrae small and elongate	**Gobies**	
	Dorsal prezygapophyses - prominent		25
25	Second knob behind neural spine		26
	No second knob		27
26	Second knob behind neural spine		
	Dorsal prezygapophysis upward pointing		
	Thick lamellar rib	**Minnow (F)**	
27	Dorsal & ventral prezygapophyses		
	- prominent	**Rocklings**	
	- not prominent		28
28	Dorsal & ventral prezygapophyses small and not prominent	**Non-rockling Gadids**	
29	Haemal spine anterior		30
	Haemal spine posterior		31
30	Dorsal prezygapophyses long and well-developed, centrum waisted	**Clingfish**	
	Heavy appearance; haemal spine has thick base	**Eel (FM)**	
31	Flattened laterally, upper and lower edges frilly		
	Thoracic vertebrae with prominent lateral processes	**Sea stickleback**	
	Edges not frilly		
			32
32	Flattened laterally, long and rectangular edges not frilly		
	Dorsal and ventral prezygapophyses long and well-developed		
	White colour (may be translucent)	**Dragonet**	
33	Dorsal prezygapophyses absent		
	Neural arch broad-based		
	Single thick lamellar rib		
	Two neural foramina		
	Spines long and back-curved	**Wrasse**	

Species characteristics

ANGUILLIDAE - Eel *Anguilla anguilla* (FM; Fig. 6)

Vertebrae

The caudal vertebrae of the eel (Fig. 6b) have a characteristic heavy appearance. The centrum is broad and square. The positions of the two spines along the centrum are very characteristic and once recognised, will prove to be a useful tool enabling quick identification of the bone. The haemal spine is **anterior** and curves backwards from a thick base. The ventral prezygapophyses are short and downward pointing. The neural spine, arising from near the **back** of the centrum, is relatively short when compared with the haemal spine. Near the base of the neural spine is a characteristic notch, below which the very small dorsal postzygapophyses are found. The dorsal prezygapophyses are also short and blunt. The centrum is characterised by a single thick lamellar rib, which can give a loose cross-like appearance, and the face of the centrum is very concave. The ventral postzygapophyses are also short.

The thoracic vertebra (Fig. 6a) is similar to the caudal in having a heavy appearance and the posterior neural spine has a thick base. In particular note the broad flat parapophyses.

The characteristic lower jaw of the eel is also shown (Fig. 6c). These bones are regularly found in spraints.

Figure 6: Eel

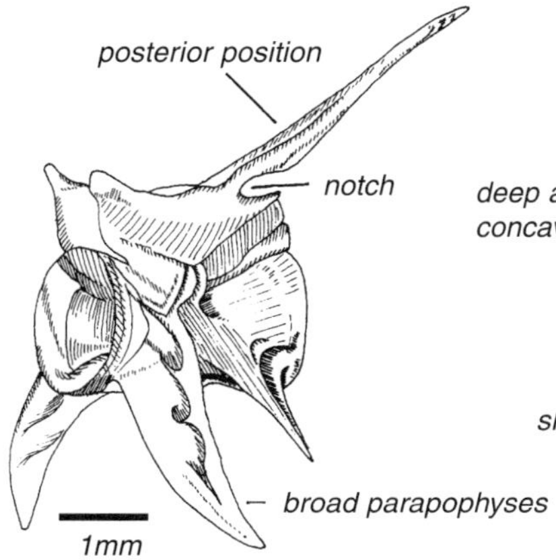

a. Eel thoracic vertebra

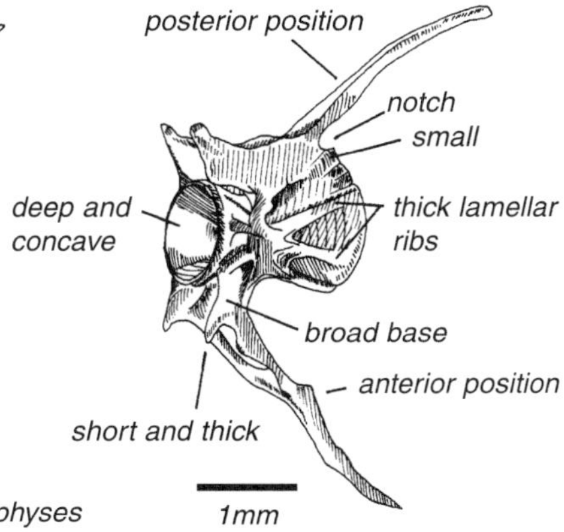

b. Eel caudal vertebra

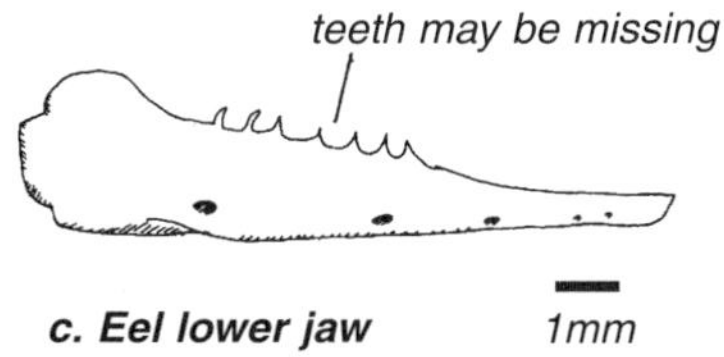

c. Eel lower jaw

Relationship to fish length:	FL = 0.90 VL + 35.63
	(Equation from Wise 1980)
Caudal vertebrae	FL = 1. 152VL + 0.92: r = 0.932
Thoracic vertebrae	FL = 1.024VL + 1.28: r = 0.970
	(Equations from Thom 1990)

SALMONIDAE - Salmonids Salmo spp. (FM; Fig. 7)

A major problem in faecal analysis has been the difficulty in telling salmon (*S. salar*) from trout (*S. trutta*) because the thoracic and caudal vertebrae are very similar. Thus, in the main key the two species are grouped together as salmonids. In this section we have detailed the bones which help identify between the two species - the atlas and premaxilla.

Figure 7: *Salmonids*

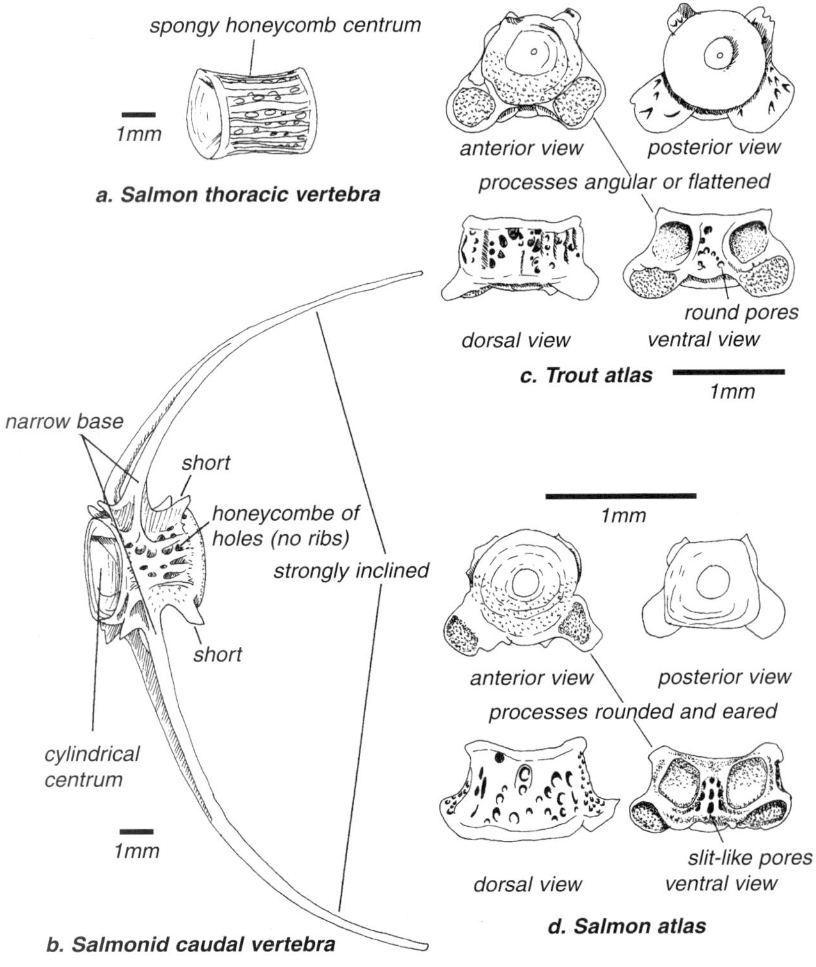

Vertebrae

Salmonid vertebrae are not strongly ossified, giving them a rough porous texture and making them particularly prone to digestion and disintegration.

1 Caudal (Fig. 7b). The centra are cylindrical and appear almost perfectly square in lateral view. There is a honeycomb pattern of holes over the centrum surface, missing only from the smooth anterior and posterior margins. The dorsal pre- and postzygapophyses are short and strongly inclined upwards; the ventral zygapophyses are angled in a similar manner. The neural and haemal spines are long, narrow and strongly back-curved. The neural and haemal arches are narrow-based and there is no neural foramen.

2 Thoracic (Fig. 7a). Thoracic vertebrae are characterised by cylindrical centra with almost square lateral views, like the caudals. There is no evidence of spines on the thoracic vertebrae, which have a honeycombed structure, but with no ridges on the lateral surfaces.

Atlas

Feltham and Marquiss (1989) found diagnostic differences between the atlas bones of trout and salmon and these descriptions of the atlases are taken from them.

The figures highlight the three diagnostic features described in the text - the shape, pores and processes. With both species, there is a degree of variability in these features, so the species is best identified using all three features.

Salmon: Salmon atlases (Fig. 7d) have no apparent waists, being short relative to the vertebral width and the dorsal portion of the ventral surface slopes outwards dorso-ventrally. The surface pores are typically slit-like (or narrowly ovate) and can be arranged in columns (particularly the pores in the dorsal region). The processes are generally eared, usually rounded but occasionally angular.

Trout: Trout atlases (Fig. 7c) appear waisted and are relatively tall when compared to the vertebral width. Pores are round (broadly ovate), often large, few in number and cover the complete surface. The processes are angular and flattened, and do not protrude as ears.

Premaxillae

Salmon: The premaxillae of salmon (Fig. 7e) are flattened laterally, triangular in shape and are approximately twice as long as they are high (cf. trout). The apex of the bone is directed postero-dorsally and is situated over the posterior half of the bone. There is a low ascending process consisting of a triangle of bone inclined postero-dorsally. From the posterior edge of this process a flange of bone runs the length of the medial surface. This flange provides attachment for the teeth, which are in a single row. There are 5-8 teeth, which are long and incurved. The lateral surface of the premaxilla often has a distinctive scaly texture. Above the tooth-bearing flange the medial surface is flat and featureless (cf. trout).

The important features of the premaxillae are their low triangular shape, height approximately half the length, and a flat medial surface.

Trout: The trout premaxilla (Fig. 7f) is like the salmon's in being laterally flattened and triangular in overall shape. It is, however, relatively taller, with its length being no more than 1.5 times its height. The dorsal apex is situated over the posterior half of the bone and is directed postero-dorsally. Anteriorly there is a low, triangular ascending process. Medially a flange of bone runs downward from the posterior edge of the ascending process, continuing caudally. As in the salmon this flange provides insertion for the single row of 6-8 teeth, which are long, conical and incurved. Above the tooth row in the centre of the medial surface there is a convex bulge of bone. This bulge is not present in the salmon's premaxilla.

The important features of the premaxillae are their high triangular shape and central bulge on the medial surface.

The characteristic salmonid lower jaw is also shown (Fig. 7g).

Relationship with fish length

Thoracic vertebrae	FL = 1.02VL– 1.02 (Equation from Wise 1980: Accuracy ±1cm) FL = 0.720VL + 1.21; r = 0.98 (Equation from Thom 1990)
Caudal vertebrae	FL = 0.751 VL + 1.93; r = 0.965 (Equation from Thom 1990)
Atlas	FL = 60.5AW - 8.95 (n = 200; rs = 0.961) (Equation from Feltham & Marquiss 1989: AW = atlas width)

Similar groups or species

Pike: Thoracic vertebrae are similar to salmonid caudals in also having no discernible processes, but can easily be distinguished from the latter by their stout lamellar ribs (not found in salmonids).

ESOCIDAE - Pike *Esox lucius* (F; Fig. 8)

Vertebrae

The vertebrae of pike (Fig. 8a) are characterised by having no spines or processes. They have a honeycombed spongy centrum, but also have prominent ribs running along their sides, giving them a very solid appearance.

The lower jaw is also shown - note the long sharp teeth (Fig. 8b).

Similar groups or species

Salmonids: Thoracic vertebrae also have no discernible processes, but can easily be distinguished from pike vertebrae by the absence of stout lamellar ribs.

Figure 7: Salmonids - continued

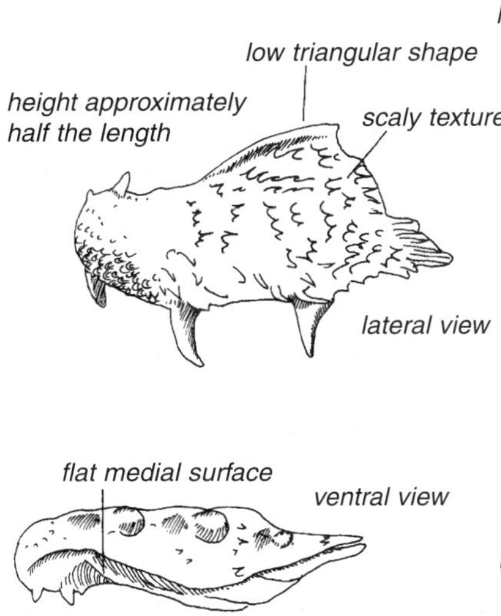

e. Salmon premaxilla 1mm

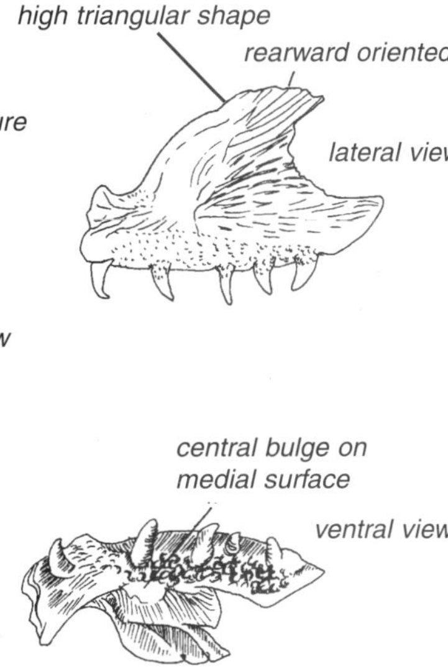

f. Trout premaxilla 1mm

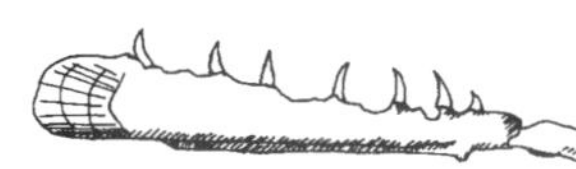

g. Trout lower jaw

Figure 8: Pike

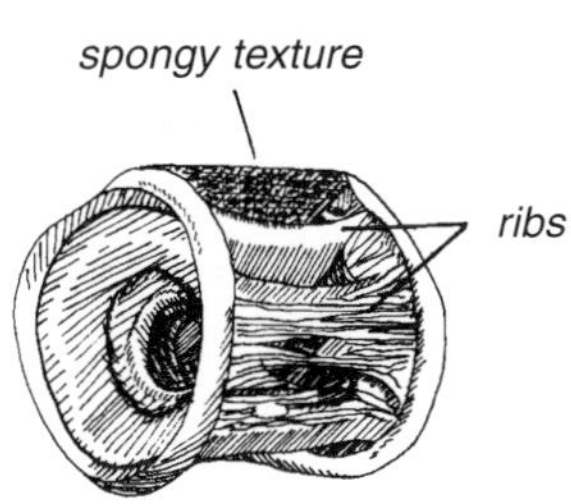

Note: no spines.

a. Pike vertebra 1mm

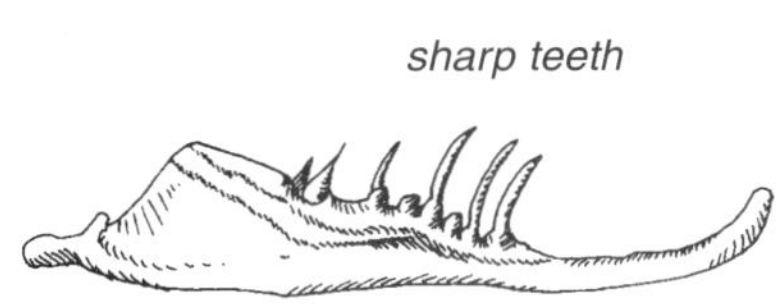

b. Pike lower jaw

CYPRINIDAE - Minnow *Phoxinus phoxinus* (F; Fig. 9)

Vertebrae

Narrow-waisted centrum with single thick prominent rib (Fig. 9a). Spines and their bases of similar length and size, both sweeping backwards beyond the rear face of the centrum. The dorsal pre- and postzygapophyses are prominent and point upwards. A characteristic feature of the minnow's vertebrae is a secondary knob behind the dorsal prezygapophyses. The ventral prezygapophyses are absent. The ventral postzygapophyses are also prominent and inclined horizontally.

Pharyngeal (gill arch)

A distinctive hook-shaped bone with up to eight blunt teeth, usually in a single row (Fig. 9b). The shape is very characteristic of the family.

Similar groups or species

Chub (*Leuciscus cephalus*), roach (*Rutilus rutilus*), rudd (*Scardinius erythrophthalmus*), gudgeon (*Gobio gobio*) and bream (*Abramis brama*): Some of these species can only be separated by an examination of the numbers and rows of their pharyngeal teeth. See Wheeler (1978, pages 102-103) for details.

Relationship with fish length

Caudal vertebrae	FL = 0.514VL + 1.27; r = 0.988
Thoracic vertebrae	FL = 0.506VL + 2.06; r = 0.984
	(Equations from Thom 1990)

Figure 9: Minnow

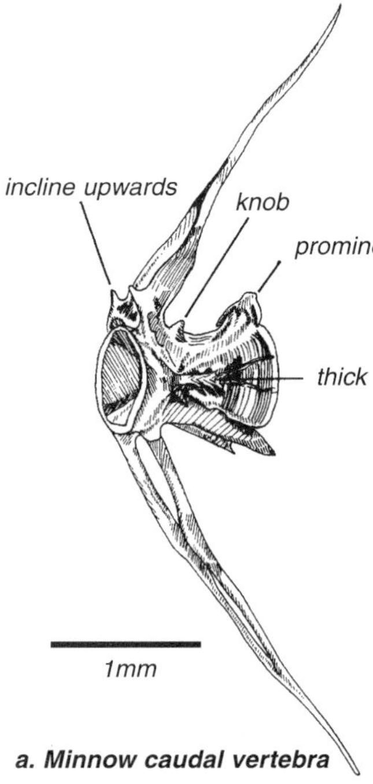

a. Minnow caudal vertebra

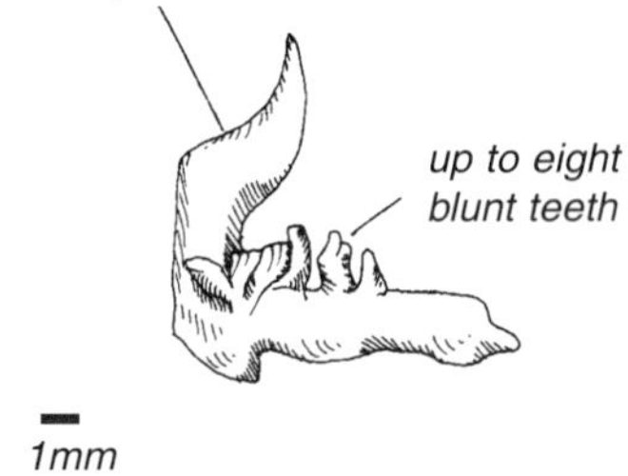

b. Minnow pharyngeal teeth

Figure 10: Stone loach

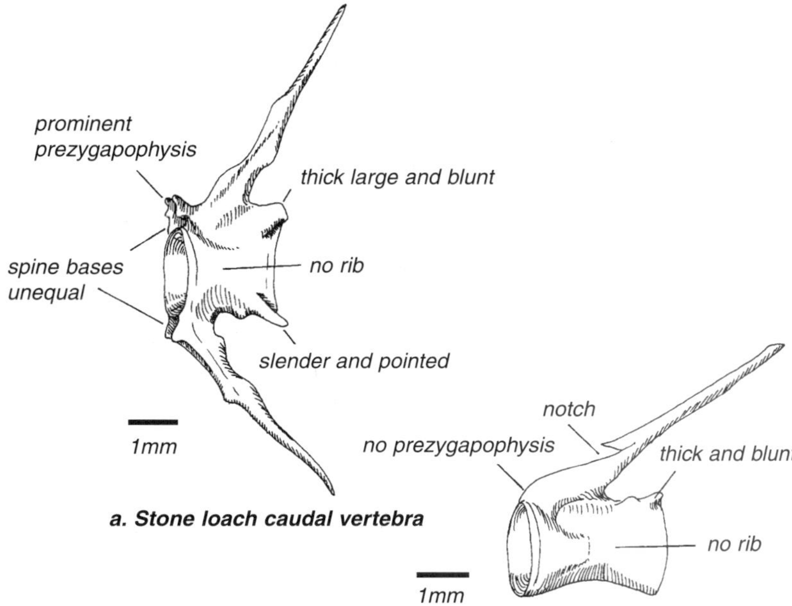

a. Stone loach caudal vertebra

b. Stone loach thoracic vertebra

COBITIDAE - Stone loach *Barbatula barbatula* (F; Fig. 10)

Vertebrae

Caudal: Centrum with no distinct rib, but possible rib markings on centrum (Fig.10a). Both spines are thick, with the dorsal one pointing more backwards than the thicker neural spine. Bases of spines are also unequal. Dorsal prezygapophyses are prominent but smaller and point sharply downwards. Dorsal postzygapophyses are thick, large and blunt, while the ventral ones are more slender and pointed.

Thoracic: Like that of the caudal vertebra, the centrum has no ribs (Fig. 10b) and the notch on the neural spine is characteristic. There are no prezygapophyses, while the dorsal postzygapophyses are thick and blunt.

Estimation of fish length

Caudal vertebrae	FL = 0.593VL + 0.51
Thoracic vertebrae	FL = 0.489VL + 0.52
	(Equations from Thom 1990)

GOBIESOCIDAE - Clingfish *Lepadogaster* spp. (M; Fig. 11)

Vertebrae

The most striking feature of clingfish vertebrae is the extreme development of the dorsal prezygapophyses, which immediately distinguishes them from those of all other species. They may be 50% or more of centrum length and are inclined slightly upwards. The centrum is rectangular and distinctly waisted, lacking any distinct ribs or sculpturing. It is usually translucent and rarely exceeds 3mm in length.

Figure 11: *Clingfish*

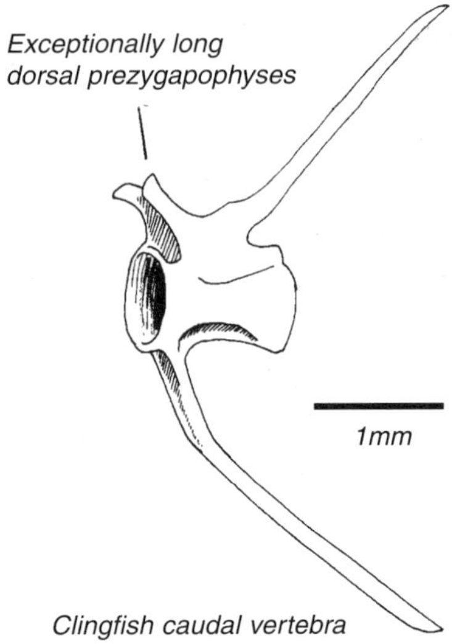

Figure 12: *Cod and Saithe*

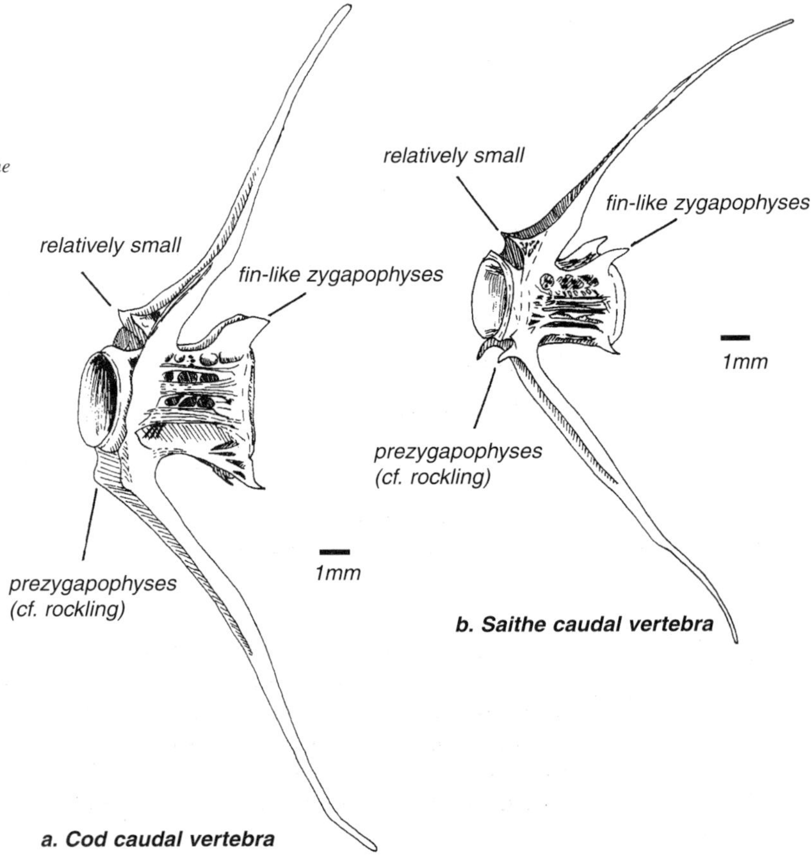

GADIDAE (M)

Non-rockling gadids (Fig. 12)

The vertebrae of the non-rockling gadids may generally be distinguished from those of rocklings by the well-developed prezygapophyses. Only very rarely do they carry the small secondary zygapophyses often found below the main dorsal prezygapophyses on rockling vertebrae.

As there are well over 20 gadid species in British waters, the vertebrae of only cod and saithe are described here. Others are detailed in Watt *et al.* (1992).

Cod *Gadus morhua* (Fig. 12 a)

Vertebrae

The centra are rather short, with their height varying from 95-106% of length. There are usually two, but up to four, distinct horizontal lines of ossification, which may form clear ridges, but these always have many interconnecting septa. These ridges are fluted posteriorly where they frequently split. The prezygapophyses are short, extending beyond the front of the centrum only in the short anterior caudal vertebrae (cf. rockling).

Relationship with fish length

log FL= 4.3523 + 0.9202 log VL (n = 26, r = 0.995),
where VL = centrum length.

Saithe *Pollachius virens* (Fig. 12 b)

Vertebrae

Saithe vertebrae are strongly waisted, the smooth anterior margin sloping steeply inwards towards the beginning of the horizontal ridging. There are generally two, occasionally three ridges, confined to near the midline, which are joined by many interconnecting septa. In some specimens these fuse to form a single raised ridge, which widens and splits behind. The prezygapophyses are narrow.

Relationship with fish length

Caudal vertebrae	FL = 57.8CL + 28.57 (n = 16, r = 0.998)
Thoracic vertebrae	FL = 0.014VL - 0.144 (n = 13, r = 0.716)
	(Equation from Grant 1984)

Note: In both rockling and non-rockling gadids the neural arch is narrow-based. There are no neural foramina because the nerves exit the arch by open areas between adjacent narrow-based arches.

Premaxillae

Cod, Saithe, Pollack *P. pollachius*, (Fig. 12 c)

The ascending process is higher than the articular, but less so than in rocklings. The two processes are separated by a shallow interprocess notch. The anterior premaxillary cleft is also shallow so that the base of the ascending process is broad - this contrasts with the premaxillae of rocklings where these two features are both deep - resulting in a distinct constriction at the base of the ascending process. The occlusal surface

Figure 12c: Saithe premaxilla

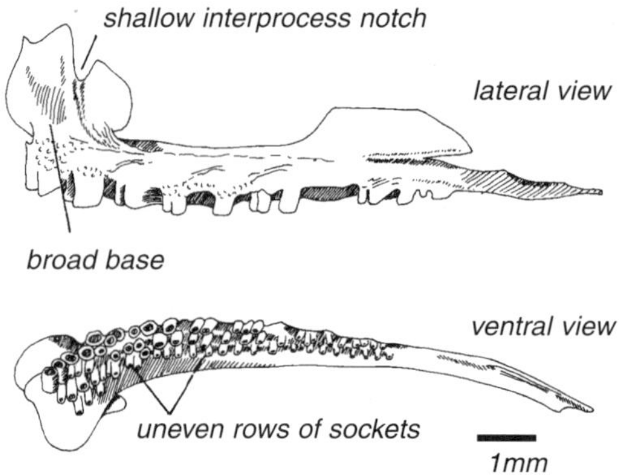

Figure 13: Rockling

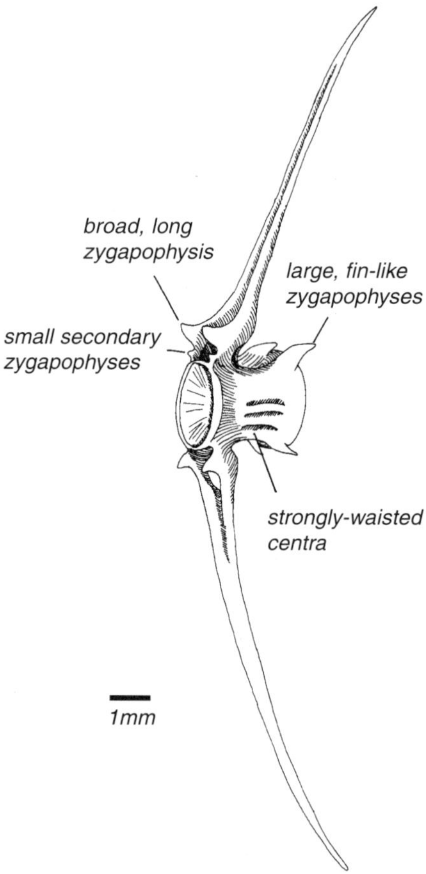

a. Five-bearded rockling caudal vertebra

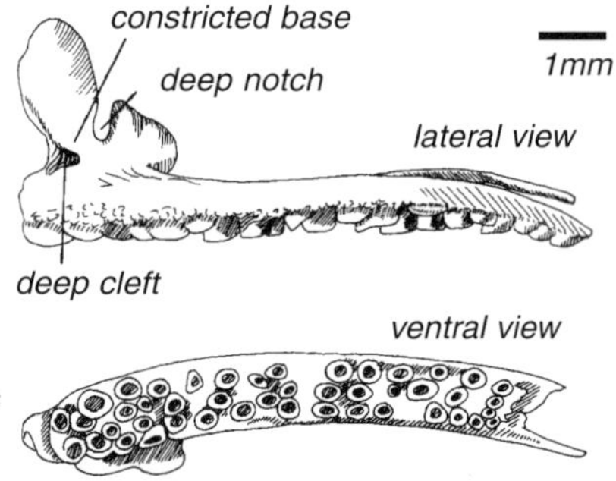

Note: occlusal surface varies between rockling species.

b. Five-bearded rockling premaxilla

bears four or more uneven rows of conical teeth, the numbers of rows depending on species and size. The teeth on the outer row are largest and in the cod they are massive. The teeth are, however, very fragile, break off easily and are unlikely to survive digestion intact.

ROCKLINGS: *Ciliata spp.* (five-bearded), *Gaidropsarus spp.* (three-bearded) and *Enchelyopus cimbrius* (four-bearded) (M; Fig. 13)

Vertebrae

Rockling vertebrae (Fig. 13a) have very large broad prezygapophyses and dorsal postzygapophyses, often extending beyond the margins of the centra. There is frequently a second short pointed dorsal prezygapophysis situated below the main zygapophysis (a feature rarely found in non-rockling gadids). The generally strongly waisted centra are typically rectangular, although those more anterior may be roughly square. The surface sculpturing on the centra varies between species:

> Northern (*C. septentrionalis*) and five-bearded rocklings: two to five low longitudinal ridges of ossification along the centra.
>
> Four-bearded rockling: Two or three well-defined lamellar ribs running close together near the middle of the centra.
>
> Three-bearded rockling: A single, broad, stout rib runs along the midline.

Watt *et al.* (1992) provide further details on rockling vertebrae, including useful photographs.

Relationship with fish length

Thoracic vertebrae	FL = 0.018VL - 0.181 (n=20, r = 0.984) (Equation from Grant 1984)

Premaxillae

In all rockling species the ascending process is considerably taller than the articular, but the most useful identification feature is the great depth of the interprocess notch and premaxillary cleft. The former reaches close to the ramus and, along with the deep anterior cleft, results in the base of the ascending process being distinctly constricted. In several species the articular process is free behind the ramus, giving its base a marked waist. The post-maxillary process is low and rectangular. The pattern of tooth sockets and relative ramus width varies between species. In five-bearded rocklings the occlusal surface is broad and flat, the tooth sockets being similar in size. In most other species the ramus is narrower and the outer socket row considerably larger.

The deep interprocess notch and anterior premaxillary cleft, resulting in the constriction of the anterior process's base, distinguishes rockling premaxillae from those other gadid species found commonly in otter spraints.

ZOARCIDAE – Eelpout or viviparous blenny *Zoarces viviparus* (M; Fig. 14)

Vertebrae

Eelpout vertebrae (Fig. 14a) are often pale turquoise or green in colour. The centrum is slightly taller than it is long. The broad base of the neural arch is also rather tall and together these two features give the bone a rectangular shape in lateral view. There is a single, strong, lamellar rib running along either side of the centrum. The concavities of the centrum are asymmetrical as in butterfish. The neural spine is very straight and roughly equal in length to the haemal spine. The haemal arch narrows uniformly from the centrum towards the haemal spine (cf. butterfish). The dorsal pre- and postzygapophyses are well developed, with only the latter extending beyond the end of the centrum. The dorsal prezygapophysis is strongly inclined upwards. In most specimens there is a small ventral prezygapophysis.

Relationship with fish length

Thoracic vertebrae $FL = 0.010VL - 0.287$ ($n=21$, $r = 0.977$)

Similar groups or species

Butterfish: In lateral view the centrum of the butterfish appears shorter and looks squarer than in the eelpout. The more anterior caudal vertebrae can be distinguished by the uniform narrowing of the haemal arch in the eelpout (no elbows). The dorsal prezygapophysis is generally inclined less strongly upwards in the butterfish, but this feature is not reliable as the degree of incline varies in both species.

Premaxillae

The most striking feature of the premaxillae (Fig. 14b) is the extremely tall columnar ascending process, which is at least twice the height of the articular process and from which it is divided by a narrow V-shaped notch (cf. butterfish). The articular process has a pointed apex. The moderately long ramus bears two or three rows of tooth sockets on its ventral surface, with the outer row being the largest. Some pleuronectids have similar premaxillae (see page 43), but those of the eelpout can be distinguished by having:

a. more rows of teeth (most pleuronectids have only one)
b. ramus which is broader than deep
c. teeth on the ventral surface of the ramus

GASTEROSTEIDAE – Three-spined stickleback *Gasterosteus aculeatus* (FM; Fig. 15)

Vertebrae

The vertebrae (Fig. 15a) have a characteristic triangular shape when viewed end on. The bones are small. The centrum is narrow-waisted, with lamellar ribs running towards the centre of the waist. The broad base of the haemal spine is usually characterised by the presence of a large hole. The neural spine is also broad-based, but is slightly shorter and not so swept back as the haemal spine. The dorsal prezygapophyses are robust and pointed. The ventral prezygapophyses are absent. The vertebrae look very shiny.

Figure 14: Eelpout

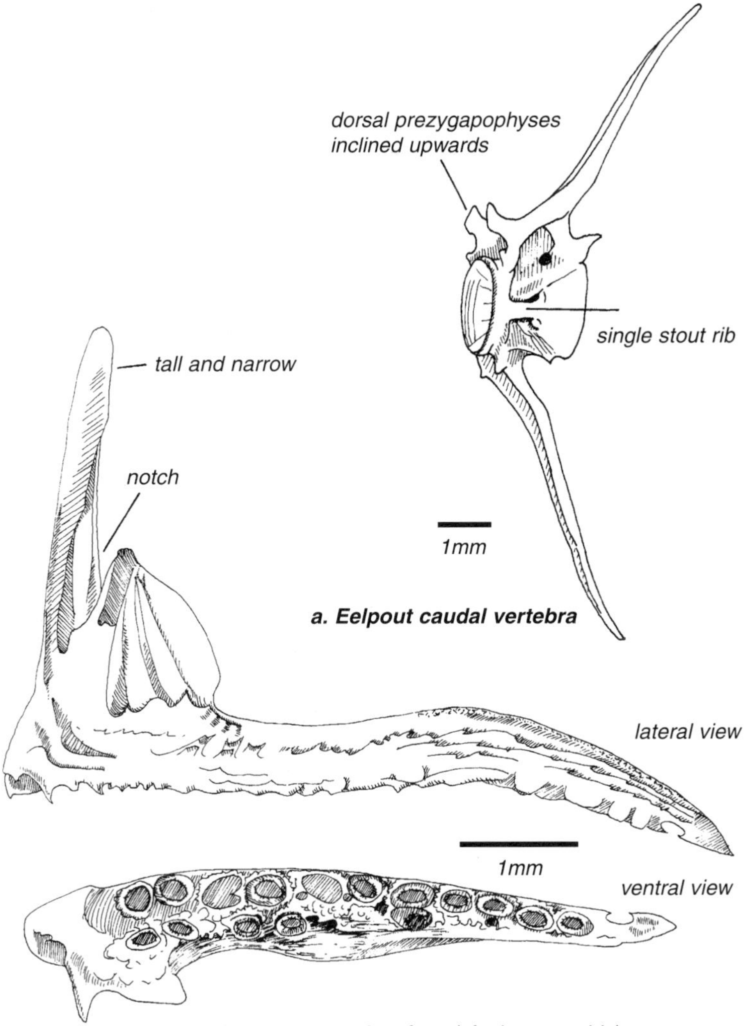

a. Eelpout caudal vertebra

Note: teeth are on ventral surface (cf. pleuronectids).

b. Eelpout premaxilla

Relationship with fish length

Caudal vertebrae	FL = 0.471 VL + 0.7
Thoracic vertebrae	FL = 0.433VL + 0.24
	(Equations from Thom 1990; no r values listed)

Sea (15-spined) stickleback *Spinachia spinachia*

Vertebrae

Caudal: The centra are flattened laterally, with a characteristic frilly edge and a definite waist (Fig. 15c). Both spines are posterior and very short, while their bases are large and flattened with large foramina.

Thoracic: The thoracic vertebrae are characterised by large lateral processes extending from a narrow-waisted centrum (Fig. 15b).

Relationship with fish length

Thoracic vertebrae   FL = 0.013VL - 0.039 (n = 11, r=0.829)
(Equation from Grant 1984)

Figure 15: Stickleback and 15-spined stickleback

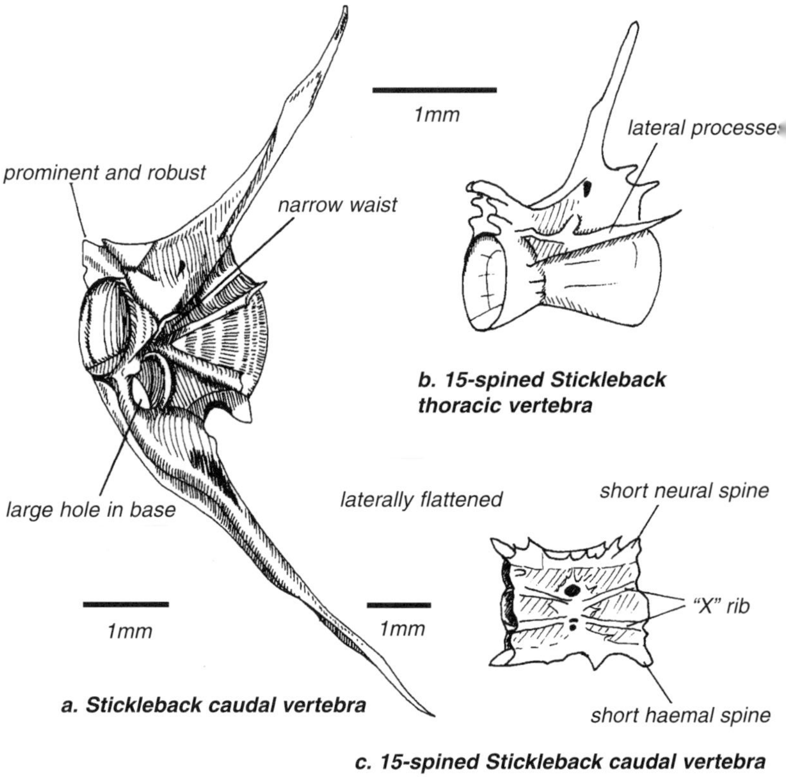

SYNGNATHIDAE – Greater pipefish *Syngnathus acus* (M; Fig. 16)

Vertebrae

Caudal: The centrum is long relative to its height and characterised by a number of foramina opening on the dorsal side (Fig. 16b). Both spines are flattened laterally and are very short and rise almost vertically from near the middle of the bone. The dorsal postzygapophyses are prominent, point upwards and can be nearly as large as the neural spine. There is no haemal arch, both spincs remaining separate and pointed. The dorsal prezygapophyses are blunt and short, but are also prominent. Both ventral zygapophyses are absent.

Thoracic: The thoracic vertebrae are similar to the caudals, but have stout lateral processes (Fig. 16a).

Figure 16: Pipefish

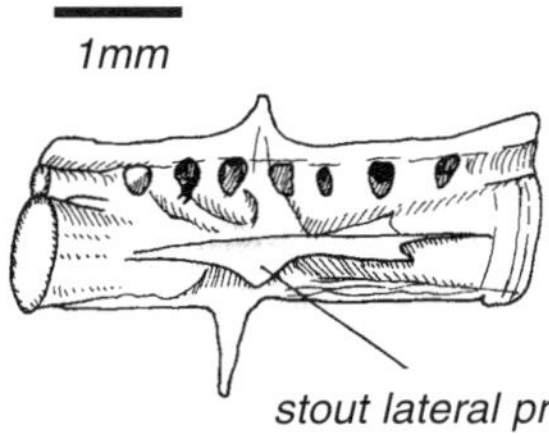

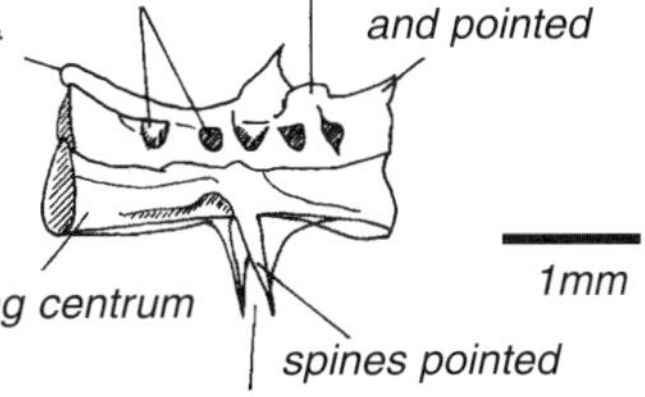

a. Pipefish thoracic vertebra *b. Pipefish caudal vertebra*

COTTIDAE - Bullrout *Myoxocephalus scorpius* and Seascorpion *Taurulus bubalis* (M; Fig. 17)

Vertebrae

Cottid caudal vertebrae (Fig. 17a) appear roughly square in lateral view. The sides of the centra are concave. In larger specimens (3mm), one or more prominent bony ridges may be present, while in small specimens the lateral surface is often featureless with no ribbing or sculpturing. The neural arch is broad-based, with its spine arising either centrally or behind the centre and often curving upwards from its base. The dorsal prezygapophyses are very prominent, extending far beyond the anterior edge of the centrum. The ventral prezygapophyses are small, but are absent in the more anterior caudal vertebrae.

Relationship with fish length:

VL is 1.4 - 1.7% FL; max. VL ca. 7mm

Premaxillae

The premaxillae of cottids are highly distinctive, having very tall anterior processes and a ramus bearing multiple rows of very small tooth sockets (Fig. 17b). The ascending process is a tall, lamellar plate of bone set across the ramus, its narrow edge orientated laterally. There is a deep dividing notch between it and the articular process, which itself is tall and roughly rectangular. The ramus has a long, strong, well-developed postmaxillary process giving it a roughly triangular appearance.

Bullhead *Cottus gobio* (M; Fig. 18)

Vertebrae

Bullhead caudal vertebrae (Fig. 18b) have a centrum with a single thick rib, and the neural spine is short and rises centrally. Haemal spine is also short, but thicker than neural spine. Base of neural spine is much larger than that of haemal spine. Dorsal prezygapophyses are large and prominent, and the ventral ones are short. Foramen in base of neural spine. Fig. 18a shows a thoracic vertebra.

Figure 17: Bullrout

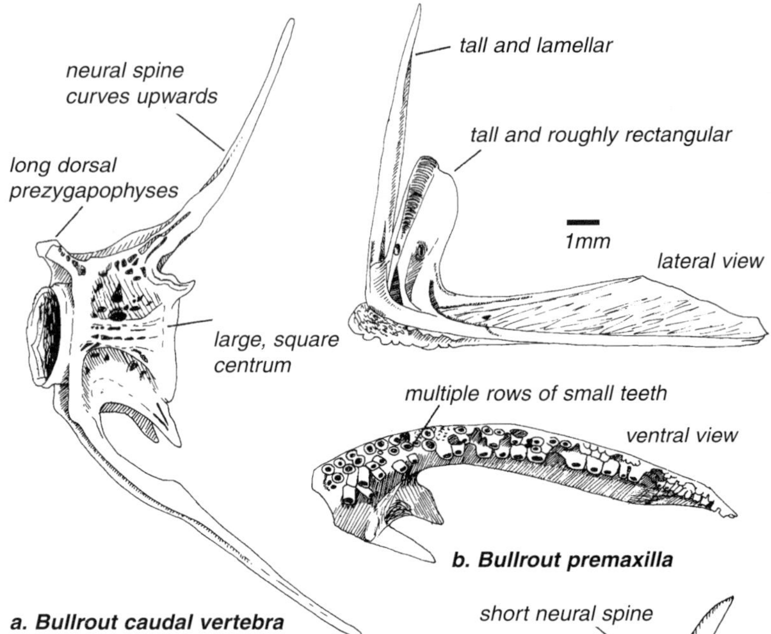

a. Bullrout caudal vertebra

b. Bullrout premaxilla

Figure 18: Bullhead

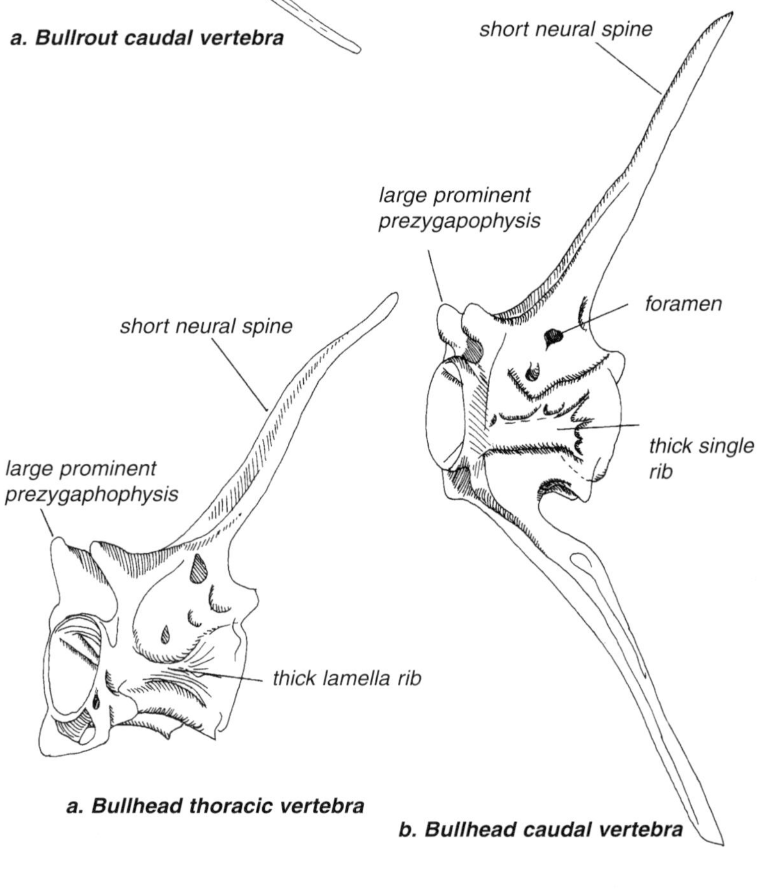

a. Bullhead thoracic vertebra

b. Bullhead caudal vertebra

CYCLOPTERIDAE (M)

Lumpsucker *Cyclopterus lumpus* (Fig. 19)

Vertebrae

The thin papery texture of lumpsucker bones distinguishes them immediately from those of all other species. Because of this lack of ossification, the bones are generally preserved poorly in spraints, being prone to breakage and digestion. The centrum is taller than it is long and bears one or two longitudinal septa along either side. The bases of the neural and haemal arches are joined anteriorly by a sheet of bone, which runs between them and inside the front edge of the centrum. A series of short septa run between this sheet of bone and the anterior edge of the centrum. There are no dorsal or ventral prezygapophyses. The neural arch is broad-based and both the haemal and neural spines are long and back-curved.

Relationship with fish length

VL is 1.7-2.3% FL;   max VL = 12.2mm

Figure 19: *Lumpsucker*

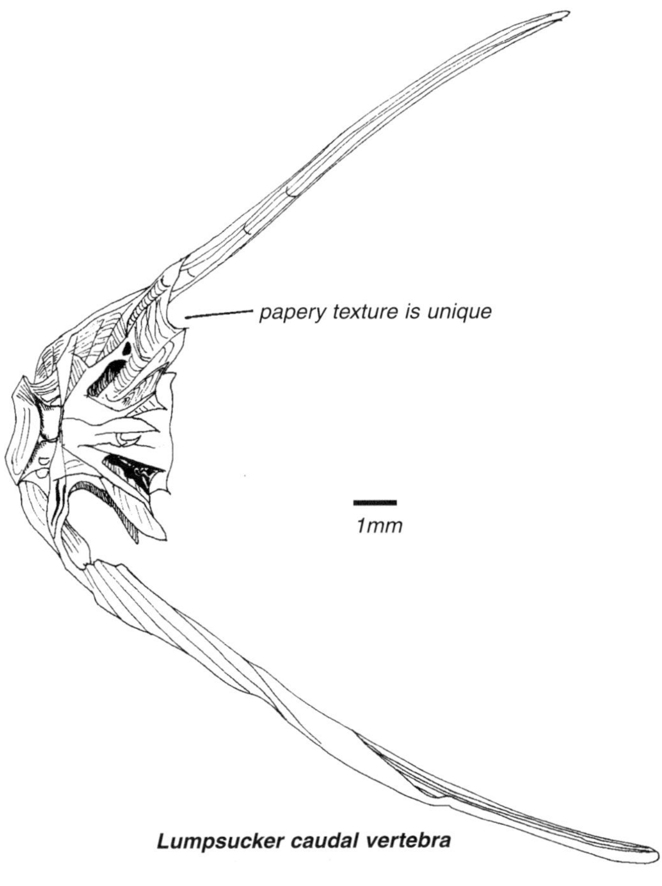

Lumpsucker caudal vertebra

Sea snails *Liparis* spp. (Fig. 20)

Vertebrae

Haemal spine much longer than neural spine, but both arise from a broad base. The anterior face of the centrum is concave. There are no prominent prezygapophyses, the dorsals being blunt and the ventrals almost non-existent. The postzygapophyses are both short and pointed. The dorsal spine usually has a single large foramen.

Figure 20: *Sea snail*

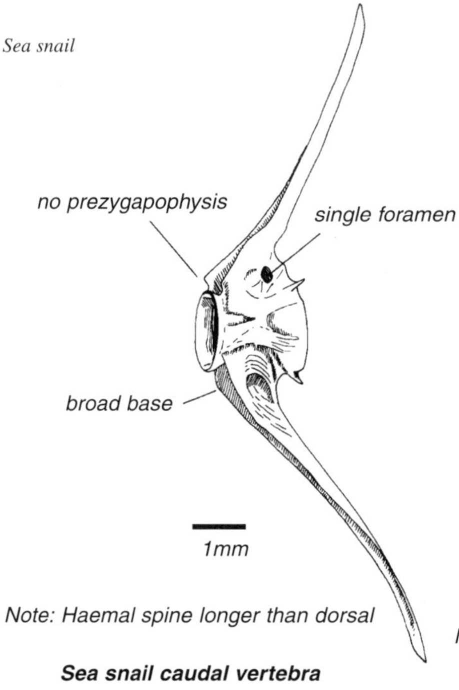

Figure 21: *Perch*

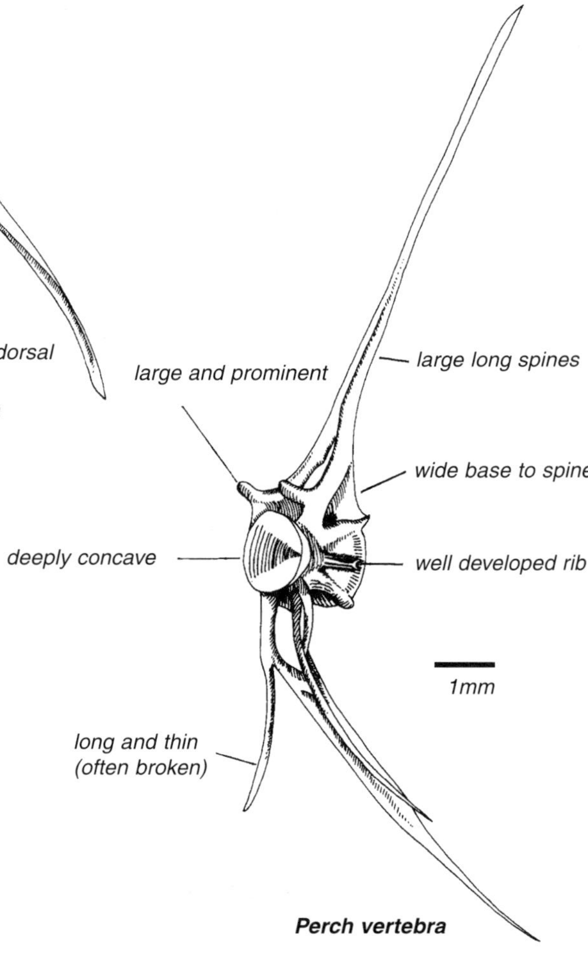

PERCIDAE - Perch *Perca fluviatilis* (F; Fig. 21)

Vertebrae The centrum is narrow-waisted with one or two well-developed ribs. The anterior face of the centrum is deeply concave. The neural spine is longer than the haemal spine, but is not so swept back. The bases of the spines are unequal, with the neural much wider than the haemal. The dorsal prezygapophyses are prominent and large, extending beyond the face of the centrum. The ventral prezygapophyses can be long and thin (but are usually broken). Dorsal postzygapophyses are pointed whereas the ventral are blunt.

Similar species Ruffe (*Gymnocephalus cernuus*), pikeperch/zander (*Stizostedion lucioperca*)

Relationship to fish length

Caudal vertebrae	FL = 0.985VL + 0.32 (r=0.985)
Thoracic vertebrae	FL = 0.531VL + 1.32 (r=0.992)
	(Equations from Thom 1990)

LABRIDAE - Wrasses (M; Fig. 22)

Vertebrae The centrum is relatively short (length no greater than height) (Fig. 22a). There are no prezygapophyses. The neural arch is broad-based and the haemal spine is anterior. The front of the bone is free of projections, making a clean curve from neural to haemal spine. There are usually two neural foramina. The ventral postzygapophyses are long and project strongly downwards, but these are prone to breakage. A most useful characteristic is the presence of a single strong lamellar rib of bone, which runs along the midline of the centrum. The neural and haemal spines are long and back-curved.

Relationship with fish length

VL is 1.5 - 2.0% FL (more posterior vertebrae are shorter)

Similar groups or species Sea snails (Cyclopteridae): Anterior caudal vertebrae (Fig. 20) have broader-based spines, while the more posterior bones have small prezygapophyses, which are not present in wrasses (see Watson 1986).

Pharyngeal teeth In wrasses the pharyngeal teeth (Fig. 22b) are highly distinctive, being very robust and remarkably persistent, so that they are often found in spraints. The short rounded teeth are arranged in irregular rows on the three-lobed bone and have probably developed in response to a diet of hard-shelled molluscs and crustaceans (Wheeler 1969).

STICHAEIDAE - Yarrell's blenny *Chirolophis ascanii* (M; Fig. 23)

Vertebrae The vertebrae (Fig. 23) bear two, occasionally three, well-defined lamellar ribs on a strongly waisted centrum. The prezygapophyses are prominent and strongly inclined upwards. The two spines are of similar length and both sweep backwards. The neural spine is central, rising from a broad

Figure 22: *Wrasse*

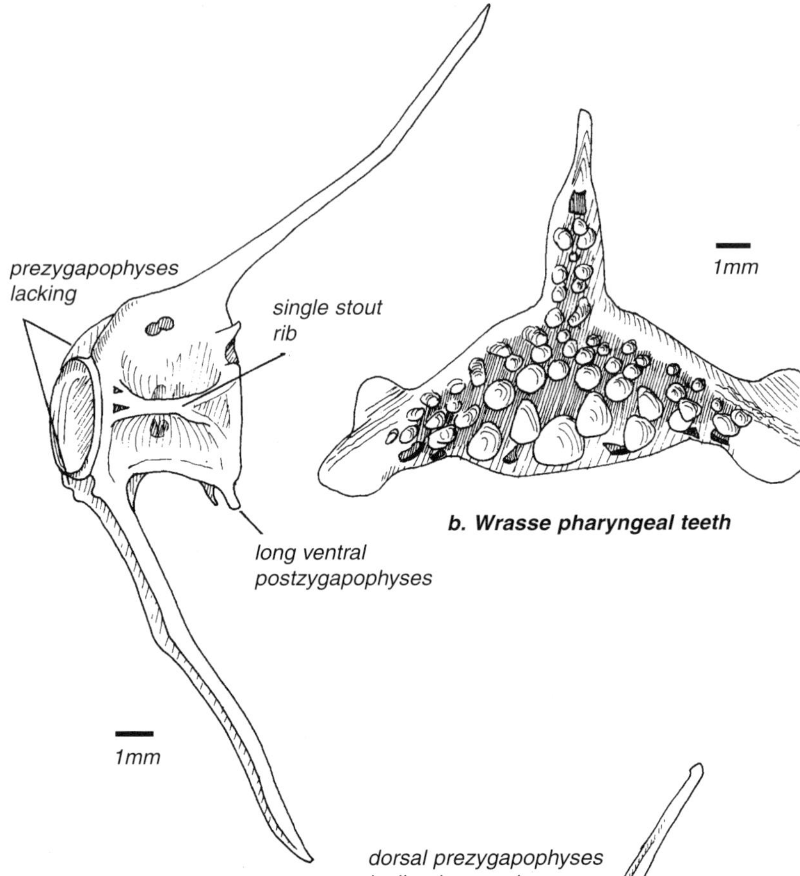

a. Wrasse caudal vertebra

Figure 23: *Yarrell's Blenny*

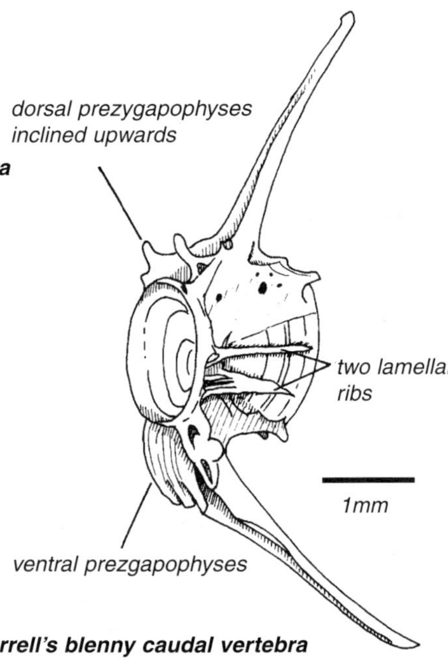

Yarrell's blenny caudal vertebra

base. The haemal spine arises towards the front of the centrum and from a less broad base. There are two neural foramina. The ventral prezygapophyses may follow the line of the haemal spine.

PHOLIDAE - Butterfish *Pholis gunnellus* (M; Fig. 24)

Vertebrae

The centrum is roughly square in profile. The anterior concavity is very shallow and the posterior one is very deep (Fig. 24a). The most distinctive feature of the centrum is the single strong rib running along either side.

Neural arch is broad-based, with a very straight neural spine, which in the more anterior vertebrae is longer than the haemal spine. The base of the haemal arch of the more anterior vertebrae flares out from the centrum before bending inwards and backwards to form the haemal spine, resulting in a distinctive elbow on the haemal arch. The dorsal prezygapophyses are inclined slightly upwards and do not extend beyond the end of the centrum. There are one or two neural foramina.

Relationship with fish length

Thoracic vertebrae   FL = 0.011VL - 0.147 (n = 20: r = 0.973)
(Equation from Grant 1984)

Similar groups or species

Eelpout (Zoarcidae): In lateral view the centrum of the eelpout appears taller and more rectangular than that of the butterfish, which appears square. The more anterior caudal vertebrae can be distinguished by the angled elbows at the base of the butterfish's haemal arch. The dorsal prezygapophysis is generally inclined less strongly in the butterfish, but this feature is not reliable.

Premaxillae

The premaxilla (Fig. 24b) is characterised by a rather short ramus and fused anterior processes. The ramus bears two rows of tooth sockets; the larger outer row extends along the entire length of the bone and the shorter inner row ends short of the rear of the bone. The ascending process is a robust column of bone, to which the articular process is entirely fused. The articular process is low and slopes downwards towards the back of the ramus.

Similar groups or species

The premaxillae can be distinguished from those of:

1. eelpouts by
   a. being shorter and squatter
   b. having only two rows of teeth
   c. having anterior processes almost completely fused together

2. gobies by
   a. relatively short ramus
   b. lack of a deep notch between the anterior processes
   c. lack of multiple rows of tooth sockets.

Figure 24: Butterfish

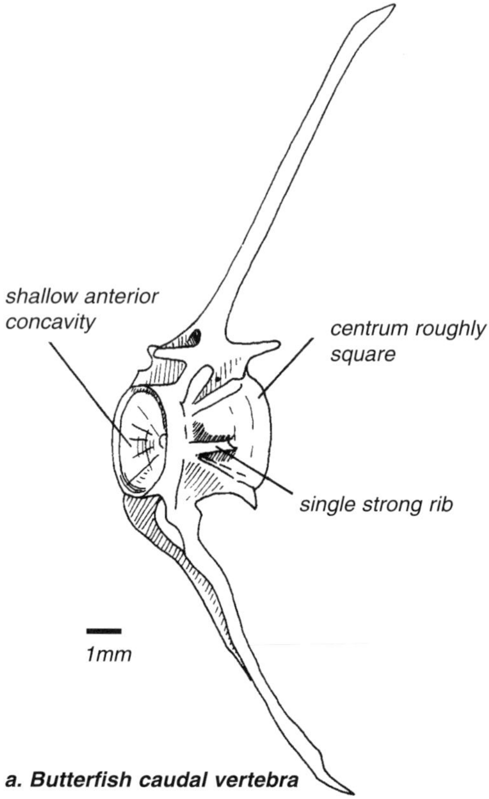

a. Butterfish caudal vertebra

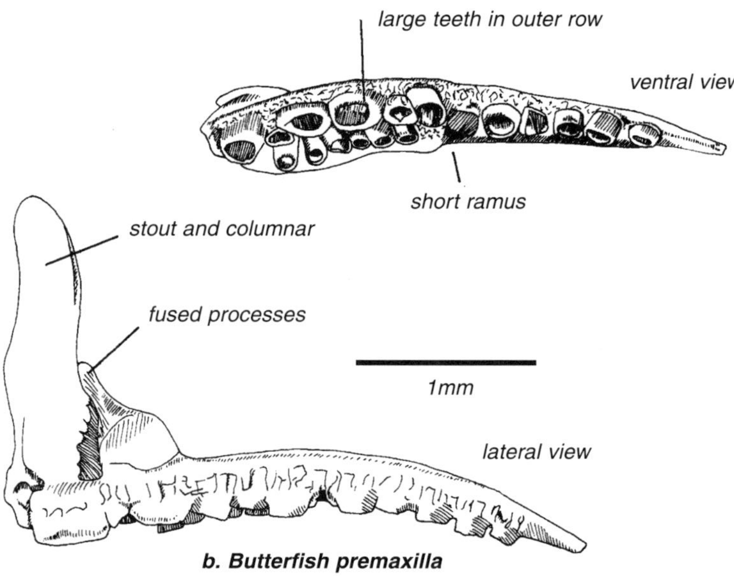

b. Butterfish premaxilla

CALLIONYMIDAE - Dragonets *Callionymus* spp. (M; Fig. 25)

Vertebrae

Dragonet vertebrae are long and rectangular, usually very white and often slightly translucent. The centra are strongly flattened laterally, particularly towards their centres where they are very narrow. Neural and haemal spines arise towards the rear of the centrum and are short blunt-ended and point backwards, lying almost parallel to one another. Both the dorsal and ventral prezygapophyses are long and well developed. There are two foramina on each lateral surface.

Relationship with fish length

VL is 2.8 - 3.3% FL
Max. VL = 10mm (more posterior vertebrae are longest and narrowest)

Similar groups or species

Scad/mackerel posterior caudal vertebrae. Dragonet vertebrae can be distinguished from these by their lateral flattening and blunt-ended neural and haemal spines.

Figure 25: *Dragonet*

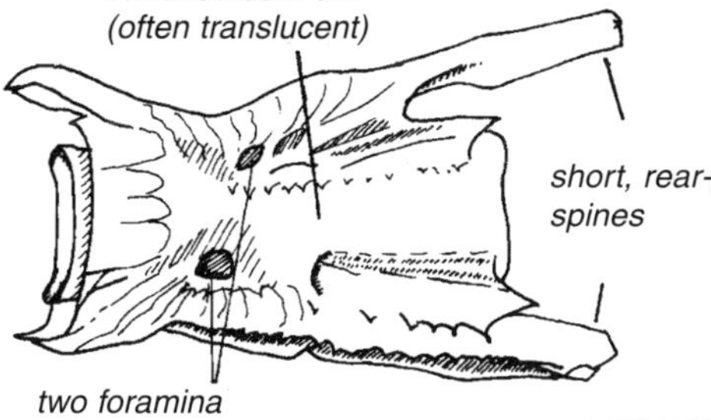

GOBIIDAE - Gobies *Gobius* spp. (M; Fig. 26)

Vertebrae

The centra are long and narrow with a very pronounced waist. They are also shiny and smooth, and free from ribs or sculpturing (Fig. 26a). Their length is 1.4 - 1.7 times their height. The neural and haemal spines arise anteriorly. In the more anterior vertebrae the neural arch is broad-based and the nerves exit via a distinct foramen. In the more posterior bones the base of the arch is shorter and there is no foramen. There are no prezygapophyses. The vertebrae are never large; commonly 1 - 2.5mm long (maximum length 3.5mm).

Relationship with fish length

VL is 1.6 to 2.1% FL

Premaxillae

The premaxillae (Fig. 26b) are characterised by a very deep interprocess notch and a relatively long ramus. On the ventral surface are several rows of tiny teeth sockets.

Figure 26: Goby

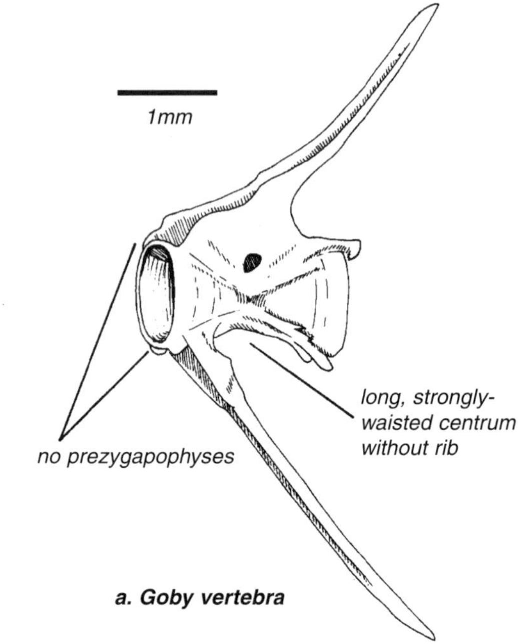

a. Goby vertebra

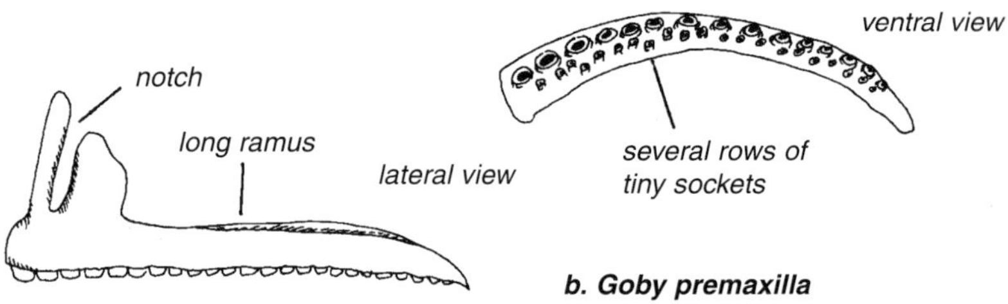

b. Goby premaxilla

PLEURONECTIDAE & BOTHIDAE (M; Fig. 27)

Flatfishes: Dab *Limanda limanda*, Plaice *Pleuronectes platessa* and Flounder *Platichthys flesus*.

Vertebrae

The most striking features of flatfish vertebrae are the very long straight neural and haemal spines, which are almost perpendicular to the centra in the more anterior caudal vertebrae (Fig. 27a). The centra are usually higher than they are long and may be hexagonal in anterior or posterior profile. Badly damaged bones can often be recognised as being from flatfish by this short hexagonal centrum. Most species bear lateral processes (apophyses) in the midline of the centrum. These may be longer on one side. The anterior and posterior zygapophyses are generally short.

The vertebrae of different species can be difficult to distinguish. If further identification is needed then a more detailed key, such as Watt *et al.* (1992), should be consulted.

Similar groups or species

Conger eels (*Conger conger*): Not described in this guide, but also have lateral apophyses on their caudal vertebrae. Their centra have 3 - 4 horizontal lamellar ribs, split by a single vertical rib, which is not found in any flatfish. Conger vertebrae have short neural and haemal spines.

Premaxillae

The premaxillae (Fig. 27c) of the flatfish most commonly taken by otters have a tall narrow ascending process and a ramus, which is deeper than it is broad. The ramus is relatively short with the ascending and articular processes being very tall and narrow. The posterior portion of the ramus is strongly decurved. There is a single row of tooth sockets (with a doubling of the row in some species). The peg-like teeth are situated along the inner surface of the bone (cf. eelpout). The left and right elements differ greatly, reflecting the overall loss of symmetry. The right premaxillae are less well developed than the left.

Left pleuronectid premaxillae can be distinguished from those of the broadly similar eelpout by having:

a. a ramus that is deeper than it is broad
b. a single row of tooth sockets
c. the teeth on the inner surface of the ramus
d. a strongly decurved posterior portion of the ramus.

SOLEIDAE - Dover sole *Solea solea* (M)

Vertebrae

The centra have a single strong thick rib along each side and are roughly round or hexagonal in anterior or posterior view (Fig. 27b). There is a single short apophysis on each side, approximately 25% of the centrum width long. These arise from the front of the rib, slightly below the midline and are strongly inclined downwards. The haemal arch is narrow-based, occupying less than 50% of the vertebra length. All the zygapophyses are well developed, with the prezygapophyses being short and usually inclined upwards in the Dover sole.

Figure 27: Dab and Sole

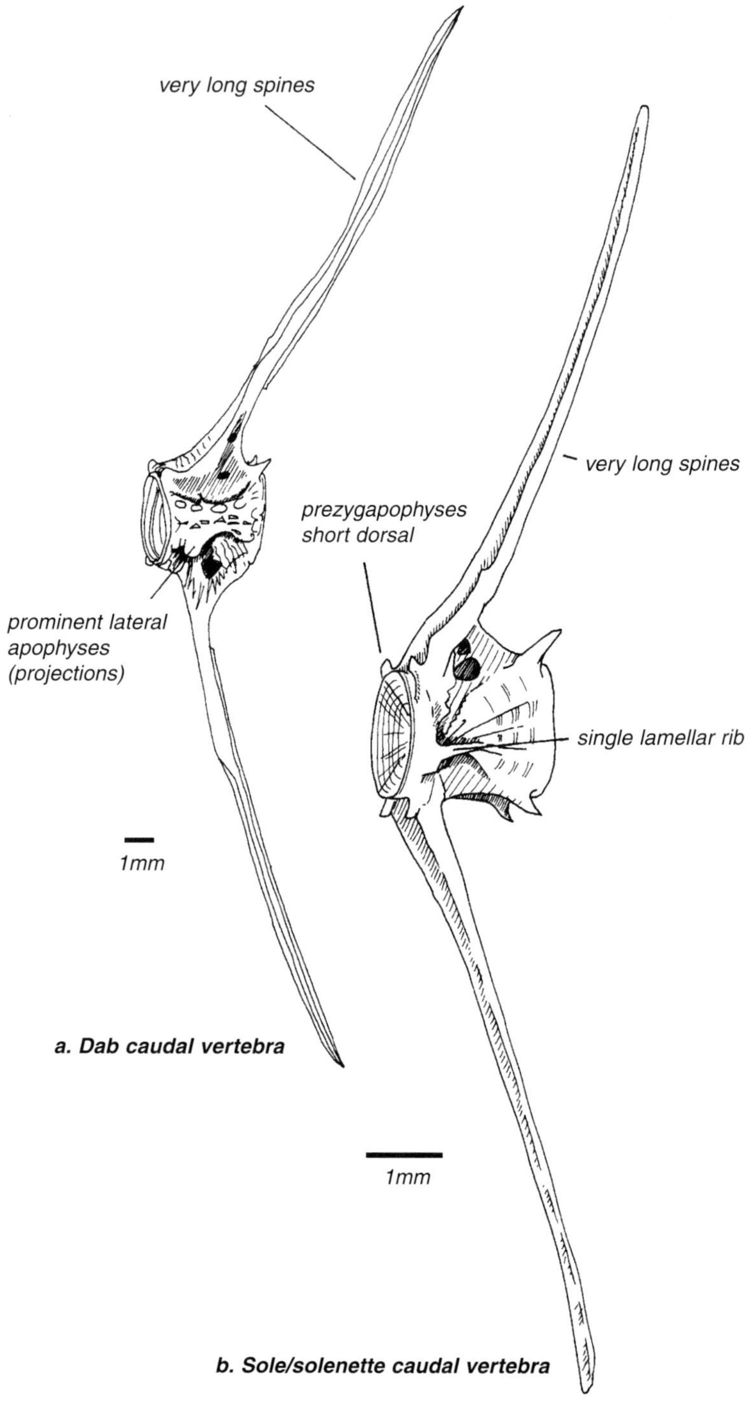

Figure 27c: *Dab and Sole - continued*

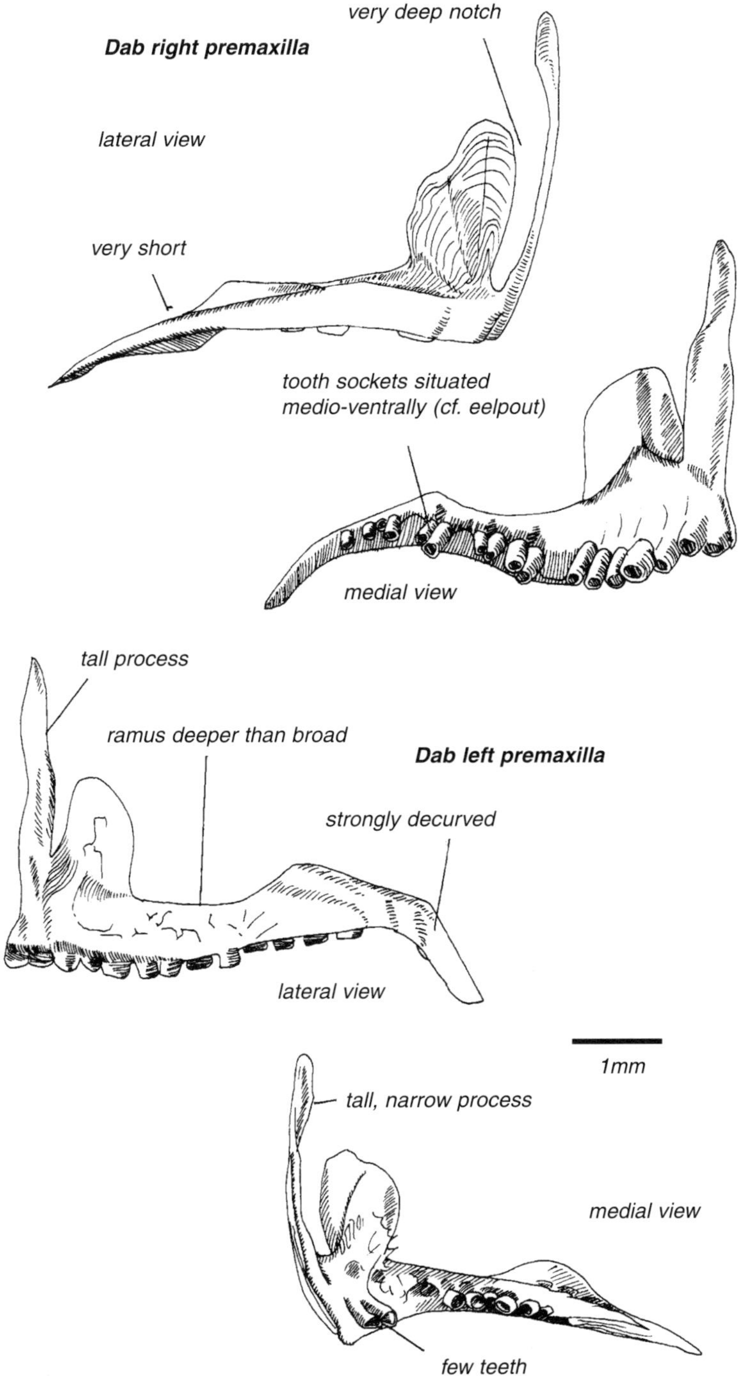

References

Brunner, H. & Coman, B.J. (1974). *The identification of mammalian hair*. Inkata Press, Melbourne.

Casteel R. W. (1976). *Fish remains in archaeology and palaeo-environmental studies.* Academic Press, London.

Chanin, P. (1985). *The natural history of otters*. Croom Helm, London.

Conroy, J.W.H. & French, D.D. (1985). *Monitoring otters in Shetland – Final report to the Shetland Oil Terminal Environmental Advisory Group.* Institute of Terrestrial Ecology. Banchory. (Unpublished).

Conroy, J.W.H. & French, D.D. (1987). The use of spraints to monitor populations of otters (*Lutra lutra L.*). *Symposium of the Zoological Society of London* 58: 247-262.

Conroy, J.W.H. & French, D.D. (1991). Seasonal patterns in sprainting behaviour of otters (*Lutra lutra L.*) in Shetland. *Habitat* 6:159-166.

Day, M.G. (1966). Identification of hair and feather remains in the gut and faeces of stoats and weasels. *Journal of Zoology*, London 148: 201-217.

Debrot, S., Fivaz,G., Mermod, C. & Weber, J.-M. (1982). *Atlas des poils de mammifères d'Europe*. Faculté des Sciences, Université de Neuchâtel, Neuchâtel (Switzerland).

Feltham, M. & Marquiss, M. (1989). The use of first vertebrae in separating and estimating the size of trout (*Salmo trutta*) and salmon (*Salmo salar*) in bone remains. *Journal of Zoology*, London 219:113-122.

Ford, E. (1937).Vertebral variation in teleostean fishes. *Journal of the Marine Biological Association*, U.K. 22:1-60.

Grant, D.A.D. (1984). *Industrial training report*. Napier College, Edinburgh.

Herfst, M.S. (1984). Habitat and food of the otter *Lutra lutra* in Shetland. *Lutra* 27: 57-70.

Izquierdo, E.R. (1988). *Contribucion al atlas osteologico de los teleosteos Ibericos*. Identario y articular. Coleccion des Estudios. Ediciones de la Universidad Autonoma de Madrid, Spain.

Jenkins, D., Walker, J.G.K. & McCowan, D. (1979). Analyses of otter (*Lutra lutra*) faeces from Deeside, N.E. Scotland. *Journal of Zoology,* London 187: 235-244.

Kruuk, H. (1995). *Wild otters predation and populations*. Oxford University Press, Oxford.

Kruuk, H., Carss, D.N. Conroy, J.W.H. & Durbin,L. (1993). Otter (*Lutra lutra* L.) numbers and fish productivity in rivers in north-east Scotland. *Symposium of the Zoological Society of London* 65:171-191.

Kruuk, H., Conroy, J.W.H. & Moorhouse, A. (1987). Seasonal reproduction, mortality and food of otters *Lutra lutra* L. in Shetland. *Symposium of the Zoological Society of London* 58: 263-278.

Kruuk, H., Conroy, J.W.H. & Moorhouse, A. (1991). Recruitment to a population of otters (*Lutra lutra*) in Shetland, in relation to food abundance. *Journal of Applied Ecology* 28: 263-278.

Kruuk, H. & Moorhouse, A. (1990). Seasonal and spatial differences in food selection by otters (*Lutra lutra*) in Shetland. *Journal of Zoology*, London 221: 621-637.

Mason, C.F. & Macdonald, S.M. (1980). The winter diet of otters (*Lutra lutra*) on a Scottish sea loch. *Journal of Zoology*, London 200: 281-283.

Mason, C.F. & Macdonald, S.M. (1986). *Otter ecology and conservation.* Cambridge University Press, Cambridge.

Miller, P.J. & Loates, M.J. (1997). *Fish of Britain and Europe.* Harper Collins, London.

Putman, R.J. (1984). Facts from faeces. *Mammal Review* 14:79-97.

Thom, T.J. (1990). *The ecology of otters* (Lutra lutra) *on the Wansbeck and Blyth river catchments in Northumberland.* M.Sc. thesis. University of Durham.

Watson, H. (1978). *Coastal otters* (Lutra lutra) *in Shetland.* Vincent Wildlife Trust, London.

Watson, H. (1986). *The feeding ecology of the European otter* (Lutra lutra L.) *in a marine environment.* M.Sc. thesis. University of Durham.

Watt, J., Pierce, G. & Boyle, P. (1992). *Guide to premaxillae and vertebrae of North Sea fish.* Department of Zoology, University of Aberdeen, Aberdeen.

Webb, J.B. (1980). *Otter spraint analysis.* Occasional Publication of The Mammal Society. The Mammal Society, Reading (out of print).

Weber, J.-M. (1989). Seasonal exploitation of amphibians by otters (*Lutra lutra*) in north-east Scotland. *Journal of Zoology*, London 220: 641-651.

Wheeler, A. (1969). *The fishes of the British Isles and north-west Europe.* Macmillan, London.

Wheeler, A. (1978). *Key to the fishes of northern Europe.* Frederick Warne & Co. Ltd, London.

Wise, M.H. (1980). The use of fish vertebrae in scats for estimating prey size of otters and mink. *Journal of Zoology*, London 192: 25-31.

Appendix 1.

Identification of Amphibians in Spraints

Amphibians can form an important part of otter diet at certain times of the year. For example Weber (1989), working in northeast Scotland, found the percentage frequency of occurrence of amphibians recorded in spraints varied from 12.9% to 47.3% with most being taken in late winter/early spring. In 150 spraints containing identifiable amphibian remains, frog (*Rana temporaria*) occurred in 146 (97.3%), while common toad (*Bufo bufo*) occurred in only four (2.7%).

There are few keys to amphibian bones. The figures of bones reproduced here are taken from Webb's original key. We would recommend that to help identify amphibian remains in spraints, a reference collection of bones be made from frog and toad - the principal bones being the vertebrae, jaw, femur and pectoral girdle.

The vertebrae are characterised by their oval shape (when viewed end on), tiny neural spine and wide processes.

Figure 28: *Frog*

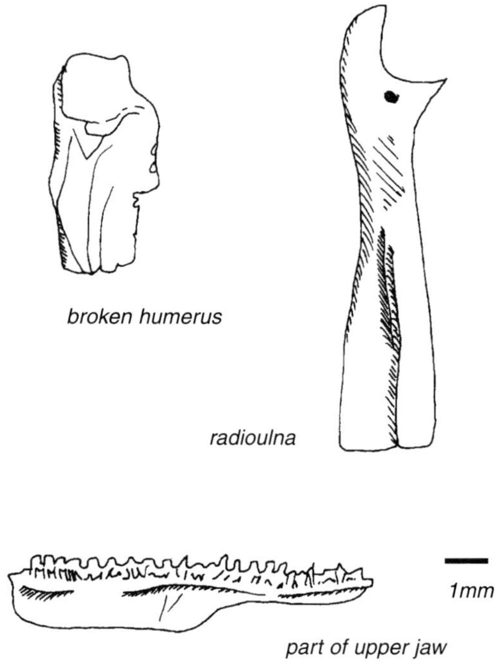

Appendix 2.

Calculation of Diet from Faecal Analysis

Both the methods used to calculate otter diet and described below will only give an index of what otters have eaten. Because different fishes have different numbers of bones (Wheeler 1969), and some bones are more prone to breakage than others (Casteel 1976), there can be no direct correlation between the numbers of bones counted in spraints and the number of fish eaten: small species with many bones will be over represented, while large prey with few bones will be under represented. At best the calculations will determine and identify the important prey in the diet.

The results of faecal analysis are usually presented as frequency of occurrence and are expressed either as;

a. Percentage Frequency of Occurrence where all the remains of each species in a spraint represent only one specimen and its frequency is calculated as the number of times it appears in all the spraints in the sample. It is calculated as:

$$\frac{\text{Number of spraints containing a particular prey species}}{\text{Total number of spraints in sample}} \times 100$$

b. Relative Frequency of Occurrence where all bones are identified for every spraint, and the frequency for each species in all spraint is determined.

The relative frequency for the whole sample is then calculated as:

$$\frac{\text{Number of occurrences of a prey item in all spraint}}{\text{Total number of all prey items identified in all spraint}} \times 100$$

Note: In (a), the sum of all the values for the whole sample should be 100.

Acknowledgements

We wish to thank the following for their help in compiling the guide - Drs Hans Kruuk and David Carss (Centre for Ecology and Hydrology) and Dr Paul Chanin (University of Exeter). We also thank Professor Peter Boyle and Dr Graham Pierce (University of Aberdeen) for allowing us to quote freely from their publication on bones of fish from the North Sea and T J Thom (University of Durham) for use of the calculations he made on fish lengths as part of his thesis. Dr Brian W Staines and Dr Mick Marquiss (CEH), Dr John Flowerdew (University of Cambridge), Gordon Woodroffe, Georgette Shearer and Vicky Harrison made valuable comments on the manuscript. Dr Roger Trout arranged for the text to be retyped and Dr Andrew Kitchener and Dr Phil Wheeler edited the text.

Getting involved - how you can help The Mammal Society

Britain is home to 60 kinds of wild mammals - found on land, in the air rivers, streams and lakes - plus another 18 seen regularly in the sea around us.

They are some of the most beautiful on Earth. They are also importan indicators of the health of our environment.

But at least half these species are under serious threat, The Mamma Society is working to change this - and with your help we can:

Join us

Membership costs from as little as £25 a year. As well as the knowledg that you are helping to safeguard the future of British wildlife you wil receive our newsletter *Mammal News* and have the opportunity to take par in a wide range of events from field trips to training weekends an seminars to conferences. There is also the opportunity to receive ou scientific journal *Mammal Review.*

Take Part

The Mammal Society relies on a committed band of volunteers to take par in mammal recording and survey work. It is only with YOUR help that w can continue with our survey and monitoring projects to conserve Britis mammals for the future.
To find out how to get involved with The Mammal Society's latest survey please e-mail **enquiries@mammal.org.uk.**

You can also join your Local Mammal Group and take part in loca mammal recording and surveying as well as participating in a wide rang of talks and events.

Make a donation!

The Mammal Society is reliant on donations for a lot of its income. Ther are many ways to donate and any donation large or small will be of grea help to our work.

For details of your Local Mammal Group and County Mamma Recorder or to join The Mammal Society or make a donatio visit **www.mammal.org.uk** or phone **020 7350 2200**.